Interviewing skills for nurses and other health care professionals

A structured approach

Robert Newell

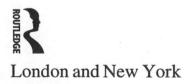

London and New York

First published 1994
by Routledge
11 New Fetter Lane, London EC4P 4EE

Simultaneously published in the USA and Canada
by Routledge
29 West 35th Street, New York, NY 10001

© 1994 Robert Newell

Typeset in Times by LaserScript, Mitcham, Surrey

Printed and bound in Great Britain by
T.J. Press (Padstow) Ltd, Padstow, Cornwall

British Library Cataloguing in Publication Data
A catalogue record for this book is available from the British Library.

Library of Congress Cataloging in Publication Data
Newell, Robert, 1954–
    Interviewing skills for nurses and other health care professionals:
    a structured approach/Robert Newell.
    p. cm.
    Includes bibliographical references and index.
    1. Medical history taking. 2. Interviewing.
    3. Nursing assessment. I. Title.
    [DNLM: 1. Interviews – methods. 2. Nursing Assessment –
    organization & administration. WY 100 N5461 1993]
    RC65.N48   1993
    616.07'51 – dc20
    DNLM/DLC
    for Library of Congress   93-10048
                                                           CIP

ISBN 0–415–07793–1 (hbk)
ISBN 0–415–07794–X (pbk)

To Caroline

Contents

Figures

1 Introduction

TOWARDS EFFECTIVE INTERVIEWING

Interviewing patients and clients is a key element of nursing practice, involving both the gathering of information and the establishment of a relationship between the participants. Without effective interviewing, it is difficult to see how nursing interventions can be successful, since both accurate information and mutual trust between nurse and patient are required. Whilst observation can offer important information, it is very often the client's own report which is the richest source. Equally, nursing interventions *can* help with very little action by the client, yet it is more likely that the client will also be required to play an active role. This in turn will be helped by the establishment of adequate rapport. Although interviewing takes up a good deal of time in nursing and other health care professions, it is, as we shall see later in this chapter, by and large done poorly. In view of this, the key issues are to recognize that there is room for improvement and to identify strategies which can help bring that improvement about. This book aims to offer such strategies, using a pragmatic, structured approach to the interviewing process. I have chosen to examine interviewing using a particular structure, the cognitive-behavioural approach, and introduce this standpoint and examine the reasons for choosing it later in this chapter. It is not, however, necessary to accept this approach, since it forms part of a more general problem-solving view of human experience which is shared by numerous other structures, including the nursing process.

It is unlikely that health care professionals intentionally interview unsympathetically, talking down to clients and ignoring their bewilderment and desire to ask questions. Equally, nurses and others probably do not deliberately ignore the large amount that is now known about the processes governing information presentation and recall. Finally, it is unimaginable that interviewers would actually *want* to undermine the client's ability to comply with instructions.

Despite this, the three key aspects of interviewing – information, emotion and behaviour change – are handled by interviewers in such a way that the client often leaves a consultation with precisely these impressions. Indeed, clients often report that their chief area of dissatisfaction during medical consultations is the clinician's poor interviewing skills (Ley, 1977). This appears to be because the clinician has a different world view from the client, which is kept a secret throughout the interview. In the view of the clinician, the client is there to answer a series of questions which enable the clinician to isolate particular areas of difficulty and 'prescribe' appropriate remedies. By contrast, the client is more likely to desire an interaction with the clinician which concerns how her particular difficulties are likely to affect her in the real world outside the consultation setting. Furthermore, the client and clinician are likely to come from worlds which are literally different: different in education, income, class, specific knowledge and vocabulary. Although it is most likely that the clinician will be advantaged in all these spheres, it is, paradoxically, the client who has to make allowances for the clinician's differing background (Dillon, 1990).

The clinician has comparatively little to lose from this mismatch in interview expectations and performance. It may well be that instructions to the client are inadequately followed by her, or that the client feels less and less able to voice concerns or ask questions in subsequent consultations. The clinician is very often unaware of these issues owing to imperfect questioning technique, and some aspects of the mismatch work to her advantage (for example by shortening interview length). The clinician is, in any case, shielded from having to consider her own shortcomings as a seeker for and provider of information by retreating behind the defence offered by the concept of the non-compliant client. Certainly, compliance with therapeutic advice is often very poor (Rachman, 1977), but I claim later that client compliance is primarily the responsibility of the clinician. However, in the early medical and nursing literature, client factors in compliance issues received far more attention than clinician factors, which have only more recently come under frequent scrutiny (Ley, 1979).

If the negative consequences of poor interviewing for the clinician are few, the consequences for the client, by contrast, are potentially grave. At its simplest level, the clinician is likely to receive inadequate or inappropriate information due to poor interviewing, with the result that any decisions made regarding the presenting problem are likely to be equally inadequate or inappropriate. Even if information is adequately gained and an accurate picture of the problem formed, poor advice-giving skills may still lead to a low level of adherence, again with potentially damaging consequences. The client may also suffer through reluctance to return to the clinician if further difficulties arise, thus delaying further intervention. More subtly, the client may come to be perceived as troublesome, unmotivated or argumentative. Such clients are likely to receive less clinician time than clients who are perceived positively by health care workers (Stockwell, 1972).

Having said that clinicians often interview clients badly, and having suggested that they do not do so deliberately, we may now ask: what *does* lead to such difficulty? Although both nurse education and medical training now place increased emphasis on acquiring specific consultation skills, these still often remain a low priority when compared with mastering skills of nursing diagnosis, performing complex manual tasks, and knowledge of core subjects like anatomy, physiology and psychology, and it has been suggested that the structure of medical training, at least, actively inhibits what interviewing skills students already possess (Helfer, 1970). Where interviewing techniques are taught it is often as part of more general education regarding interpersonal skills and self-awareness, as reflected by the blurring of these distinctions in many textbooks. Furthermore, there is often a lack of opportunity to practise such skills in a safe and reflective environment where risk-taking is permissible. Once the student nurse is involved in 'practising' such skills in the ward setting, it is often too late and too threatening to experiment with different interviewing styles. It is also unlikely that the ward atmosphere will be sufficiently calm and supportive to allow quiet reflection on the practice of interviewing. From this point on, the nurse is, to a large degree, 'on her own' (Birch, 1979). I mentioned above one tactic people might use to protect themselves from the consequences of their lack of interviewing skill – the client is non-compliant. There are others: 'not enough time', 'poor facilities', 'too many distractions', 'client is unintelligent', 'client has social problems', 'it's all right in theory', and so on. No doubt many of these things are sometimes true, but even in such situations, a competent interviewer will do better than a less skilled one. The difficulty is that, in the clinical setting, the nurse often has no access to either the guidance or the support which will allow her to tease out those aspects of a situation which are within her control from those which are not. More significantly, as the nurse develops these inappropriate coping tactics, in a genuine effort to understand the difficulties and complexities of the relationship of the interview, she may develop habits of behaviour and thinking which maintain the problematic interviewing style intact. Specifically, she may stay, as we all tend to, with what is familiar about her performance, regard difficulties with that performance as being due to external circumstances, and believe there are no problems with her interviewing to be modified.

It is precisely these kinds of issue that this book seeks to explore. This is a 'how-to-do-it' book, and I will discuss later how to use it in that way, but it is more than that, too. I hope not only to describe good practice, but also to demonstrate *why* it is good, referring to examples from the psychology literature relating to social skills, attitude maintenance and change, person perception and learning theories where relevant. By so doing, a framework is offered for coping with interviews and improving interviewing technique, a means of investigating your current interviewing practice (through examination of the case history material and comparison with your own interviews) and (via the suggested further reading) a source of ideas for continuing the exploration of the interviewing process.

There will be times, reading the following chapters, when you will wonder what all the fuss is about, since some of the material will seem very obvious. This is fine: I make no great claims to originality, and there is no doubt that you will already be using some of the strategies suggested. I do claim, however, that the information we examine together will be so organized that it will enable you to identify and enhance those skills you have, whilst adding others. Equally, there will, I hope, be times when you will recognize errors and problems in your interviewing, as a result of what you will read here. The only real mistake in interviewing, and it is a common one, is to assume that there are no such errors and problems.

EDUCATION AND COMPLIANCE ISSUES

I introduced earlier the notion of client 'compliance' and will retain this term because of its currency in much of the interviewing literature. The term is not, however, used here to mean passive acceptance of advice, but consenting and comprehending adherence to such advice. In Chapter 6, we shall look in some detail at issues surrounding client education and compliance with health care advice. However, because this area is so important to practice, I shall introduce it briefly at this point. There seem to be two issues which may give rise to confusion, particularly to the interviewer with a background in traditional counselling.

First, nurses are often taught to avoid advising the client directly, particularly where personal problems are concerned. This is because advice is thought to be problematic for (at least) the following reasons:

Advice prevents the client from identifying and pursuing her own chosen course of action.
Advice blocks the client from exploring emotional issues.
Advice protects the clinician from feelings of inadequacy.
Advice leads to premature closure of debate.
Advice allows the possibility of manipulation of the clinician by the client (Sundeen *et al.*, 1986).

Furthermore, some schools of thought in counselling even deny the usefulness of asking questions of the client at all, usually claiming that the chief role of the interviewer is in facilitating the client in coming to her own solutions to her problems, by the use of verbal statements and non-verbal behaviours indicative of warmth, genuineness and empathy with the client. Questions are seen as impeding this process (Rogers, 1951). Despite these possible pitfalls, cognitive-behaviour therapists routinely offer a great deal of advice, and ask a great many questions. Indeed, one form of cognitive-behaviour therapy (rational-emotive therapy) consists almost entirely of questions (Ellis, 1962). Yet cognitive-behaviour therapy, based almost entirely on interviewing and resulting interventions, has the most reliable outcome record of any of the various psychotherapeutic methods (Rachman & Wilson, 1980). The approach to interviewing examined in this book is based on the cognitive-behavioural approach to human experience, and involves applying the principles of conditioning and social learning theory (Bandura, 1977a) and investigations of the interaction of emotions, thoughts and actions to the alleviation of human distress. It is outlined briefly later in this chapter, and again, in some detail, in Chapter 4.

Thus there appears to be a contradiction between a good deal of current teaching of nurses and the cognitive-behavioural approach. I contend that this contradiction is only apparent, and may be resolved in three ways. First, there are differences in the language used to describe particular approaches. By advice, I do not mean the uncritical offering of general tactics, regardless of personal circumstances. Nor do I mean telling people what they *should* do. Cognitive-behaviourists see advice-giving as an interactive, changing process of negotiation between client and therapist, in which both strive to find the best course of action, with the therapist using specialist knowledge to offer specific information which the client can apply to the process of trying to cope. This may involve straight-forward, didactic information-giving, at one extreme, or helping the client to examine their personal feelings and circumstances through unstructured reflection, at the other. In short, advice-giving, for the cognitive-behaviourist, is any tactic which seeks to offer the client skills to use in confronting and con-quering their difficulties. Clearly there are more and less effective methods of offering such skills. Advice has a bad name in health care circles, I contend, because of poor delivery methods.

Second, it turns out that some of the assertions made by counselling orthodoxy are unlikely to be true. There is, for example, little clear evidence to demonstrate that Rogers' (1957) 'necessary and sufficient conditions' for effective therapy (warmth, empathy and genuineness) are either necessary or sufficient (e.g. Lambert *et al.*, 1978). They are certainly useful, and much of the information offered in this book both assumes that the interviewer possesses these character-istics, and tries to offer assistance in demonstrating them. In the absence of concrete information-giving, however, there are situations in which the client is unlikely ever to come to conclusions which are likely to offer the best problem-solving strategies without some sort of external guidance.

Finally, some of the assumptions which cognitive-behaviour therapy makes about clients, and which are described below, protect the interviewer from making the kind of errors commonly associated with advice-giving. Particularly important are the emphases on uniqueness, sincerity, coping ability and responsi-bility of the client. These assumptions help to strengthen the interviewer's commitment to equality between the participants in the interview, and decrease the likelihood that advice-giving will ever become simply telling the client what to do.

A second, related difficulty concerns the view that the health educator needs only to make information available in order to ensure compliance. This mis-conception seems to be a consequence both of the extremely laudable view that clients want to do what is best for them and of the underlying assumption that the motivated client will change her behaviour provided that she has access to information which will demonstrate to her how to do so.

Whilst cognitive-behaviourists strongly agree with both these views (as may be noted from the series of assumptions about the client listed below), they also recognize that they are oversimplifications. Clients may have competing needs, only some of which are compatible with either acceptance of the information offered or compliance. They may be unable to see the advantages in compliance if information is presented in a way which does not address their individual circumstances. Furthermore, even if they do not experience these competing needs, and do recognize the benefits of compliance, even the most compliant clients may have difficulties if the advice given fails to take account of their individual circumstances.

Such difficulty is simply another way of *only* telling a client what to do. Skilled interviewers recognize a client as truly having access to appropriate information only if that client has received such information in a way which relates directly to her individual circumstances, which highlights the benefits of compliance whilst identifying the difficulties, and which offers individually tailored strategies for putting the information into practice to effect behaviour change.

INTERVIEWING AND MODELS OF NURSING

Much of the above emphasis on individualized care will no doubt seem familiar to nurses who are experienced in using the nursing process in conjunction with a particular model of nursing. Indeed, much of this book is organized along nursing process lines. Thus, the book moves from assessment, through planning and implementation, to evaluation. I argue that the proper understanding and imple-mentation of strategies which enhance interviewing skill will lead to an increase in excellence of carrying out the stages of the nursing process. The imple-mentation of the nursing process through the care delivery system of primary nursing is a particular example of highly individualized care where good inter-viewing is a necessity.

Excellence in interviewing may also contribute to excellence in the use of nursing models, and the use of the interviewing framework offered in this book with nursing models is addressed in Chapter 4. However, the use of any particular model of nursing over any other is not endorsed, since I argue that none has received sufficient research support in any given settings to justify such preference. I am also unsure as to the wisdom of describing such conceptualizations of nursing as 'models' at all, since this invites comparison with the use of the word in other disciplines, where it is usually associated with tests of the model against aspects of the real world which it attempts to describe.

In nursing, such tests are rare, and, indeed, some elements of models are so constructed as to defy testing. Much as Macguire (1989) has stated with regard to primary nursing, the crucial issues concerning nursing models are those of accurate specification of what the use of a particular model is supposed to achieve, construction of reliable and valid measures to indicate whether such achievement occurs, definition of criteria according to which we can say that this achievement either has or has not occurred, and the conducting of practice-based outcome research studies using such clearly stated aims, measures and criteria. Until such conditions are met, I prefer, along with a number of other commentators, to speak of nursing 'frameworks', 'approaches', 'ideologies' or 'beliefs' (Clarke, 1987).

Having said this, it is clear that some conceptualization of what nursing is about is important, as a guide to practice. The approach I have taken throughout reflects this. Nurses will, in their different clinical situations, be using a variety of different nursing models and nursing care delivery systems. Therefore, without opting for any particular model or care delivery system, an interview approach is offered which is sufficiently flexible to allow the interviewer to use it with any such model or system.

THE COGNITIVE-BEHAVIOURAL APPROACH TO INTERVIEWING

I have noted that this book does not explicitly tie its accounts of the interviewing process to any single model of nursing. Nevertheless, I do acknowledge the importance to my thinking of one particular model of human experience and performance, and its associated system of psychotherapy. This model, the cognitive-behavioural (CB) approach, approximates to a number of models of nursing (most notably those of Johnson, 1968, and King, 1971), but is a broader account of humanity. It takes its ideas from a wide range of schools of thought in the social and natural sciences, and is itself composed of a number of differing trends which share commonalities but also vary in the details of how they account for human experience and behaviour. Above all, it is an accessible and a research-based explanation of human (and animal!) experience generally, and more particularly, of human problems and methods of addressing them. Apart from my own background in cognitive-behaviour therapy, I have used the cognitive-behavioural framework for two reasons. First, cognitive-behaviour therapy is a highly flexible approach capable of broad applications (Barker, 1982). Second, it has given rise to a range of interventions which are the best investigated and best validated in the psychotherapy literature (e.g. Kendall & Hollon, 1979). Thus, it is hoped that the cognitive-behavioural model offers the clinician a range of interviewing tactics which are not only applicable across a wide range of situations, but which are also based on the best available current data, and therefore most likely to lead to successful interviewing.

It is not necessary to accept many of the assumptions made by this model in order to benefit from its findings. Actually, the only assumption which needs to be accepted is that experimental and clinical research can tell us something useful about the way humans operate, since it is upon this kind of research that most cognitive-behavioural formulations of human thought, behaviour and emotion are based.

Nevertheless, a brief account of some of the underlying assumptions of the cognitive-behavioural approach may help when we go on to examine the implications of this approach for interviewing, by orientating you to some of the background to the ideas I am hoping to put across. Although the approach is relatively recent, dating back only 15–20 years, it has antecedents in behaviourism, humanism, information processing theory, and even psychoanalysis, dating back to the early years of this century (Newell & Dryden, 1991). The clearest of these links is with behaviourism, and with its associated therapeutic strategy, behaviour therapy or behaviour modification. Strict behaviourism stresses the importance of rewards and punishments in the outside world to the exclusion of underlying processes such as thought. Even by the late 1950s, however, it was becoming apparent that behaviourism, with its insistence on the study only of observable behaviour, was an insufficiently powerful model to explain many aspects of human experience.

In particular, the acceptance of Bandura's work on social learning theory (Bandura, 1977a) led to significant modifications to behaviourist theories and to behaviour therapy. Social learning theory states that a behaviour does not need to be directly rewarded in order for it to increase in frequency. Instead, it is enough to observe another person being rewarded for that behaviour, after which the observer will tend to carry out the behaviour also, in anticipation of reward. The importance of this for behaviourism is that it is extremely unlikely that such observational learning can occur without internal representations of reality, such as thoughts. The associated technique in therapy, modelling, was a relatively early cognitive addition to behaviour therapy. Bandura has offered further modifications of behavioural accounts, stressing the importance of 'self-efficacy' (Bandura, 1977b). According to Bandura, people are more likely to carry out a particular behaviour if they believe they are capable of so doing. The availability of reward and the person's actual capabilities are secondary to the person's perception of these two factors. Again, the important modification to behaviourism is the insistence on the primary nature of the person's internal perceptions of reality, in terms both of reward and of ability to obtain the reward.

Quite separately, therapists were working on formulations of client difficulties which emphasized thought as the central feature controlling such problems. According to cognitive therapists, human difficulties are characterized by particular patterns of thinking, which mediate disordered mood and behaviour. If these patterns of thinking can be challenged and changed by the client, the difficulties will improve (Beck, 1976). Although these formulations began from observation of clients and their characteristic thinking patterns, more recent accounts have been built on complex information-processing descriptions of human cognition, and have received considerable support in the experimental studies of non-client subjects (Williams *et al.*, 1988).

The social learning and information processing accounts of human difficulties both seem one-dimensional, but came together in the cognitive-behavioural approach. In some senses, this is hardly surprising, since the work of Bandura had invited cognition into behaviour therapy relatively early in its development. Furthermore, the cognitive and behavioural perspectives were united by more things than those which separated them, particularly with regard to therapy. Both stressed the need for rigorous evaluation of the effectiveness of the techniques they employed and both drew on experimental work from academic psychology. Both shared a common view of the genesis and maintenance of client difficulties. Although one emphasized cognition, and the other stressed the importance of behaviour, both agreed that difficulties were caused by faulty learning of one kind or another. Moreover, problematic behaviours, emotions and thoughts were not seen as being different in kind from non-problematic ones – both were primarily the result of learning.

This led to similar ideas about the nature of treatment, which was seen essentially as a process of acquisition of appropriate skills. In cognitive-behaviour therapy, the client is seen as a highly active partner in care, rather than a passive recipient. As part of this emphasis, cognitive-behaviour therapists pursue a humanistic approach which is based on the uniqueness of each individual's interaction with the environment. Consequently, cognitive-behaviourists avoid the use of diagnostic categories, looking instead at each individual's profile when planning and negotiating care (Newell & Dryden, 1991). Again, we see parallels both with the nursing process and with many nursing models.

This emphasis on human uniqueness, together with familiarity with the psychology literature on such issues as information transmission and treatment compliance, led cognitive-behaviour therapists to look closely at the interviewing process. Although early behaviour therapy was generally carried out with the therapist present, cognitive-behaviour therapy today relies, to a large extent, on the client's unsupervised efforts in combating her own difficulties. Here the importance of appropriate interviewing is paramount, since the therapist must rely on the client for accurate information regarding both her difficulties and her efforts to combat them away from the clinic, and the client must rely on the therapist to provide applicable and understandable tactics to aid her in these efforts. Thus cognitive-behaviour therapists have long recognized the need to pay careful attention to improving information-gathering, information-offering and compliance-enhancing techniques. That they have been successful is suggested by the wealth of evidence of successful therapeutic outcome and client satisfaction with the interventions offered (Rachman & Wilson, 1980).

Finally, because of their insistence both on the uniqueness of individual experience and the continuity between problematic and non-problematic behaviour, cognitive-behaviourists are also concerned both to 'normalize' the interview and to recognize its uniqueness. The interview should be as normal as possible for the client, in that it should approximate as far as possible to her experiences of social discourse in daily life, so that she experiences as little distraction from the business in hand as is practicable. On the other hand, the interviewer needs to realize that the situation is, by its nature, unique to both participants, and that both may, in consequence, need to use special skills to permit free flow of information. Both need to *work* to render the interview 'normal'.

I have talked at length about cognitive-behaviour therapy for four reasons. First, to set the scene for much of the information which will follow, since much of this information is based on the cognitive-behavioural approach to interviewing, which in turn is based on cognitive-behavioural theories and therapy. Second, to suggest that much of this information has a sound research basis. Third, because one particular cognitive-behavioural approach to assessment, which has been designed for use in a wide variety of clinical situations, will be used in the chapters on assessment interviewing (Marks, 1986). Finally, to introduce you to a number of assumptions made about humans (and, by implication, clients) by the cognitive-behavioural tradition. I shall now examine these assumptions in slightly more detail.

ASSUMPTIONS ABOUT THE CLIENT

Most of these assumptions are based on a humanistic account of human experience which emphasises the person's interaction with the environment, rather than placing her at the mercy of it. Because of this view of humanity, cognitive-behaviourists use the following set of presuppositions about clients in the interview situation.

Each client is unique

Clients have individual stories to tell, and it is the individual elements of their stories which enable clinicians to construct and negotiate interventions with clients in such a way as to maximize the likelihood of compliance and improvement. Although this may seem obvious, it is already a radical departure from a great deal of medical and nursing practice, as diagnostic categories assume very minor importance, and *general* social and personal circumstances are also not emphasized. By contrast *specific* individual social, physical, cognitive and behavioural circumstances are regarded as the most important elements in mediating change. Individual problem definition is heavily emphasized.

Each client has skills

Clients have rich lives, only small parts of which are concerned with their problems. During assessment and therapeutic interviews, these skills can be brought to bear in a number of ways, to enhance information-gathering, emotion-handling, advice-giving and compliance-generation. Furthermore, clients can bring these areas of skill to bear upon their difficulties. The interviewer can either aid or impede this process.

Each client interacts with the environment

Clients have lives away from the interview, which affect them and which they affect, about which we know very little. The more we can find out about those elements of their lives which relate to the interview, the more likely that the interview will be successful in terms of aiding the client.

Clients are like us

Largely speaking, the same sources of influence operate in our lives and those of clients. As a result, there is a strong possibility that we can form therapeutic alliances with them, and can understand and empathize with their difficulties. There is an equally strong possibility that there is nothing 'abnormal' about their behaviour, in its context. Clients are also our equals, since they resemble us in every respect other than those small areas of their lives which are problematic. Even in these areas, there reactions are similar to our own, so the equality extends into the problematic areas. I prefer the words 'consumer' or 'customer' to both 'client' and 'patient', since both the latter imply dependence. However, 'client' is retained for reasons of familiarity and because I recognize that my preferred choices are also not without their drawbacks.

Clients are honest

Until proved otherwise, it is a poor tactic to suspect that clients are wilfully concealing information. Most likely they are just waiting for the right question, statement or context. By and large they are giving us the best information they can, although there may well be occasions when they do not have access to the kind of information we seek. In such situations, we would do well to devise tactics to support their recall.

Each client sincerely desires success

Clients do not deliberately sabotage their own treatment, however simple or difficult that treatment may be. Such a notion (like the notion of the dishonest client) is a way for clinicians to defend themselves from the results of their own errors, or their own need for success at any cost, when clients do not do well. Clients do, however, experience many difficulties in complying with treatment instructions, partly because of aspects of the interview (such as those identified above) and because of issues about themselves and their environment outside the interview, of which the interviewer may either be ignorant or which she may have failed to consider.

Each client shares responsibility with the interviewer

The client has *some* responsibility for the successful outcome of any interview. However, the greater part of this responsibility is the interviewer's, since she has greater familiarity with the situation, greater power in it and (hopefully) more appropriate training in how to perform in it.

Clients desire interaction and negotiation

People generally experience social contact as of primary importance, and seek understanding of those situations with a view to attaining appropriate control. Therefore, clients make assessments of clinicians' social skills and respond accordingly. They also try to extract from clinicians the meaning of their remarks, whether these be questions or instructions, and to act accordingly when they believe these questions and instructions to have value. Where there are difficulties in extracting such meaning, they may (particularly in the face of poor social skills) seek to act according to some meaning which was not present in the original remarks. If no negotiation is forthcoming from the clinician, clients may well negotiate within themselves and act accordingly.

Each client knows what the problem is

Clients are generally well aware of the key issues surrounding their difficulties, particularly where extensive life handicaps are involved. The interviewer does not need to go on a hunt for mysterious causes, but need only listen carefully to what the client says.

Each client knows when success has occurred

Clients are generally the best judges of whether a particular intervention has or has not been successful. When their own health goals have been met, it is usually redundant, and could be counterproductive, for the interviewer to persist. The interviewer would do well to accept that client goals and interviewer goals may differ and may change.

Although it may seem obvious that the ten statements given here are very wide generalizations indeed, it is suggested that you read this book on the assumption that they *are always the case*. Ideally, you will eventually proceed through real interviews on the same assumption. The rationale behind this suggestion is that, as has been suggested earlier, it is very easy to generate rationalizations for difficulties in interviews. It is, therefore, possible that these will creep in unbidden to redress the balance away from my possibly overoptimistic assumptions about clients. There are usually tactics which yield better results than deliberately departing from the above assumptions.

As an example, let us consider the client, usually described as suffering from anorexia nervosa, on a bedrest and refeeding regime in a general hospital. Typically, these clients are perceived and described by nurses and doctors as hostile and uncooperative (Russell, 1981). On this basis, it seems obvious that Assumptions 5 and 6 cannot apply. The client is neither honest, nor does she desire success. Unfortunately, if we accept either of these assertions, then we must also assume that negotiation is impossible, and that our only course of action is to treat the client against her will. Equally unfortunately, such interventions are not only of dubious moral status, but also of extremely doubtful effectiveness (Fairburn & Cooper, 1989). By contrast, if we assert that our original assumptions about the client remain true, then we are in a position to reassess our treatment options. To begin with we may redefine goals in conjunction with the client, albeit accepting that these may, initially, be unsatisfactory to us. We could, for example, examine the life handicaps consequent upon low weight, and construct goals related to these rather than related to weight gain. At the very least, we could address these issues as well as the issue of weight gain. In so doing, we offer the client the chance to become honest and successful.

THE NURSE AS HEALTH EDUCATOR AND CHANGE AGENT

Throughout this book, the words 'nurse' and 'clinician' are used interchangeably.

Much of the information here is highly applicable to other health care staff, and a good percentage of the health care research material from which examples have been drawn relates to health care groups other than nurses. Nevertheless, it is to nurses that this book is primarily directed. Nurses are the largest group of clinical health care professionals, and spend a large percentage of their time in direct clinical contact. These facts alone would render their training in appropriate interviewing skills of paramount importance, since they are, therefore, the health workers most likely to be encountered by clients.

Thus, they have a crucial role in client education. This need not be formal health care education, but may also be informal 'education' of the client into her role in health care interactions. If the nurse repeatedly conveys to the client messages which suggest, for instance, that questioning is inappropriate, then the client becomes less likely to ask questions on subsequent occasions. Similarly, if the nurse creates the impression that passivity is expected, the client is less likely to expect to play an active role in care, and less likely to comply with instructions, since the importance of her own role has been diminished. By contrast, the client is likely to learn from the nurse's encouragement of participation in care that negotiation and compliance are important parts of treatment and recovery.

Further issues which add to the need for improved interviewing by nurses are the extended training and clinical role of the nurse. Nurses are expected to do more, and to do it to a higher level of competence than ever before in this country, and assume increasingly high levels of professional autonomy. As a result of this, they will need increasingly high-quality information upon which to base nursing-needs assessments and evaluate nursing interventions. The modern emphasis on individualized care highlights this need for accurate information. Furthermore, as the nursing role extends, we can expect nurses to assume sole care for an increasing number of clients, and, therefore, to be placed in an increasing number of formal interviewing situations. These new roles are ones which nurses are ideally placed to fill, given their domination of health care numbers and in-creasingly high levels of education. It is important that their levels of skill in interviewing rise to meet this challenge.

USING THIS BOOK

I suggest that those things which hold true for clients must also hold true for interviewers, and, as a result, emphasize the need to use this book interactively. First, the book should be *read* interactively. I strongly suggest that you stop repeatedly throughout the text and examine the assumptions and suggestions I make, attempting to reflect on your own interviewing practice to see how they fit. Second, the book should be *used* interactively. The suggestions should ideally be put into practice as soon as possible in the interviewing situation, with the aim of integrating them into your current practice. Begin to evaluate your interviews right now, using the self-evaluation tool I have given (Appendix 1) or one of your own devising. Then, as you add different elements to your interviewing, you will be in a position to keep track of the improvements.

I have also attempted to so arrange the book as to make assimilation of the information presented as easy as possible, since it is most likely that you will use the information presented if you have it readily available in memory, and that this itself is most likely if the material is presented in a way which makes maximum possible use of what we know about effective presentation of information for recall. Therefore, I try to present information in as unambiguous, clearly related a form as possible. For example, I try to describe aspects of interviewing at those points in the interviewing process where they are most likely to occur, in the hope that they will be best remembered in such settings.

Complex interviewer behaviours are broken down into simple ones wherever possible. For example, unexpectedly, there is no single section of this book entitled 'counselling clients' even though we might reasonably think that aspects of counselling would occupy a good deal of interviewing time. Although there is a pragmatic reason for this omission, in that counselling is a vast subject, there are also structural reasons, in that I see counselling as comprising a great many different activities, not all of which are done at the same time (or even by the same counsellors). As a result, aspects of this complex set of behaviours are addressed in the text (for example, when considering negotiation, goal-setting, supporting) but are viewed from the standpoint of interviewing generally, rather than therapeutic interviewing or counselling specifically.

Individuals may initially read through the book from start to finish, but it is also possible to extract relevant information from various sections of the book in any order, given some understanding of the way in which it is organized. This is part of the process of interactive use which I suggested above. In this way, I hope you will return to it again and again as a source of guidance for practice. By all means use this book as a reader and a resource, too, but primarily use it as an aid to your own expert practice and reflection. It is this latter use of the book which I primarily intend. I suggest particularly its use, either with individuals or in groups, as part of a programme of practical tuition in interviewing skills.

EXERCISES

1   Consider the last time you interviewed a client, no matter how brief or apparently trivial the interaction.

What information did you wish to gain or convey?
What was the emotional tone of the interaction?
What behaviour change was desired by you and the client?
How well did you deal with each of these issues?
What could you have done differently?

2   Read again the section on assumptions about the client.

Take each assumption in turn and try to think of an example from your clinical experience which seems to contradict it (such as the example I gave of the anorexic client). Write down each example.

Examine each example again, trying to resolve the apparent contradiction so that the assumption still makes sense.
How will the negotiation of care differ if the assumption is (a) rejected; (b) accepted?

A NOTE ON GENDER

With the exception of some of the case history material, I use the female personal pronoun throughout, as a reflection of nursing as a predominantly female profession and of women as the greater consumers of health care.

FURTHER READING

Dillon, J.T. (1990) *The Practice of Questioning.* London. Routledge.
Marks, I.M. (1986) *Behavioural Psychotherapy: The Maudsley Pocket Book of Clinical Management.* Bristol. Wright.

2 Opening an interview

BEGINNINGS – THE RUDIMENTS OF INTERVIEWING

To begin our examination of skilled interviewing, this chapter looks at that crucial time in relationships with clients when ground rules are laid for conduct of later interactions during subsequent meetings. 'First impressions count' is a truism, and it is perhaps because of the familiarity of this phrase that the importance of first meetings with clients is often overlooked. This is particularly unfortunate, both because we all take so many lasting impressions away from first meetings and the first moments of these meetings, and because, as we shall see in this chapter, this aspect of the interview is the most easily studied and improved upon by interviewers.

Imagine that the interview is like a game of chess (albeit, hopefully, without the adversarial aspects!), in which the two participants come progressively to a greater understanding of each other. Characteristically, the chess 'opening' is extensively studied by players, because it is crucial to what comes after, but also because its variables are so well defined as to render it capable of extremely formal study. A certain amount may be known about the opponent, for example through study of her earlier games, but her behaviour in *the game to come* is completely unknown. However, the possibilities in the opening are sufficiently finite to enable each player to predict, with reasonable certainty, the kinds of moves which are likely to be made by the other. It is this constrained formality which makes the opening that aspect of chess at which computers particularly excel.

So with the interview. The interviewer usually knows only a small amount about the interviewee, through referral data or communication with the referral agent or with other colleagues. Nevertheless, there will be certain constants which can reasonably be predicted from interview to interview, which the interviewer can study repeatedly, with the aim of finely honing the skills associated with starting interviews. Such repeated practice pays the added dividend of addressing one of the most important aspects of the interview. Examination of the 'opening' of the interview offers clinicians (particularly relatively inexperienced interviewers) a relatively structured experience in which to practise aspects of performance which will enhance such performance for relatively little input. It is not surprising, therefore, that Goldberg *et al.* (1984), in a study of the tuition of interviewing skills to psychiatrists, found that those aspects of interviewing which concerned openings were the most effectively learnt. Participants in the teaching programme were most significantly different from a control group with regard to such initial aspects of the interview.

Conversely, inattention to these opening aspects will be very likely to lead to great difficulty with grasping the nature of effective interviewing as a whole. To return to the analogy of chess, apparently even master players find study and play of the 'middle game' particularly difficult and uncertain. If we add to this uncertainty some flaw related to the opening, the game is often lost. In an interview, we should recognise that client impressions of us are generally formed within minutes of commencing the interview (Thompson, 1984a). If I have studied the comparatively uncomplicated aspects of beginning interviews inadequately, the amount to be lost is out of all proportion to the effort required in studying it effectively. Clients who form an unfavourable impression of me, because I make them anxious, appear distant, do not orient them to the material to follow, do not organize my conduct of the session, and so on, are then less likely to see any reason for offering useful information or complying with any instructions I may offer. Given the comparative ease of studying interview openings, these difficulties are little more than my just desserts.

It follows, then, that this chapter should be relatively uncomplicated and yet require and repay careful attention. Hopefully all these things are so, for this chapter, through the process of orienting the interviewer to the most general aspects of beginning interviews, also aims to introduce a number of issues which should be absorbed and put into practice when considering the more focal material of Chapters 4 and 5.

Within the context of opening interviews, some general themes are also explored, many of which are continued throughout this book. The opening of the interview provides here a simple introduction to what become increasingly complex issues as the interview progresses. Thus, issues to do with roles of the interviewer and client, planning the conduct of the interview and setting aims and objectives are all considered for the first time below, and repeatedly returned to in the following chapters. These issues are important at all stages of the interviewing process, and consideration of them during interview openings will provide a template for the reader to examine them again in later stages of the interview.

BEFORE THE INTERVIEW – PLANNING EACH ENCOUNTER

Earlier in this chapter, I compared the interview with the chess game, and remarked how chess experts will repeatedly examine familiar elements of the chess game and also consider the previous games of forthcoming opponents. Pre-interview strategies in the interview process are the equivalent of this stage in the chess game. There are a number of things, before being faced with the unknown interviewee, that the skilled interviewer can achieve by way of preparation.

The overall aim here is to aid the interviewer by removing as many imponderables as possible, and helping her to organize her conduct of the interview. The more organized the interview, before beginning, the less anxiety the interviewer is likely to face, and the better will be her chance of demonstrating to the client that professional competence which will most likely be associated with the client being able to cooperate in offering accurate information and carrying out negotiated therapeutic instructions (Korsch *et al.*, 1968). In other words, the more organized the pre-interview tactics, the more confident the interviewer, the greater the possibility for therapeutic trust by the client.

TIMING

It is important to attend for interviews punctually and to allow sufficient time for the interview itself, for pre-planning and for post-interview activities. This is a general case management issue which health professionals overlook. We are all familiar with the hurried and harried GP who is looking at case notes as the client walks into the consulting room, and reading those of the next client as the current one leaves. Good interviewing is impossible without good general case management. Therefore, interviewers need to ask themselves whether they are seeing too many clients on a given day, or over their entire caseload, and resist the temptation to respond to internal or external pressure to see more. Failure to do so is likely to result in hurried preparation and an ever-worsening backlog of appointments. Furthermore, the service offered to each client is likely to be lessened in quality, and many of the recommendations in this book are likely to become impossible, since, for example, it will be impossible to give clients adequate time to develop their accounts of their difficulties or to ask questions when the nurse is herself under constant pressure to 'process' clients within unrealistic time constraints. Although pressure of work is inevitable in NHS settings, the pressured clinician might usefully consider the balance between quality and quantity of consultations. GPs see many clients each day, yet the quality of such consultations is notoriously bad (Maguire, 1979). Moreover, many of these are repeat consultations, and it is worth considering how many of these would be required if adequate information had been gained and transmitted during the first such interview. One satisfied client who does not return and require further intervention is a great deal better use of time than the infinite repetition of unsuccessful interventions with the same core group of unsatisfied and inadequately handled clients, and successful interventions repay the investment made in terms of clinician esteem, client satisfaction and, ultimately caseload size, for a given service.

Successful interviewers also consider the amount of time available for the interview as part of the context within which aims and objectives are arrived at. Can the interviewer reasonably expect to achieve anything within the given time constraints, and if so, what? Clearly, this issue is connected to that of appropriate and assertive case management. In an ideal world, there is always abundant time to do everything one would want within a given interview. In reality, things are less simple. Emergency interviews will always occur, when chance or minimally planned interactions with clients take place and must be handled by the clinician. Furthermore, constraints of client and nurse attention mean that 'perfect' interviews are not unlimited in duration, but are of a length which optimizes the potential for an appropriate attention level from both.

AIMS AND OBJECTIVES

Both before and after reading referral information, the interviewer can gain from a consideration of aims and objectives. Aims refer to broad statements of interviewer intent, whilst objectives are narrower, and may generally refer to both interviewer and interviewee behaviour at the end of the interview (Jarvis & Gibson, 1985). Additionally, the interviewer may have process, or expressive, objectives, which state what kinds of experience the interviewee will have during the course of the interview (Popham *et al.*, 1969). Before reading referral data, the interviewer may consider those general aims and objectives which are true of all interviews (see exercises), and these considerations may be further specified to the current interview after consideration of such referral information. In this way, the interviewer goes into the interview with a number of ideas about what she hopes to achieve, providing direction and structure for the encounter. Making a brief note of these *tentative* suggestions about interview process and outcome before the interview will help to keep structure (Phillips, 1977), although the need for flexibility in selecting and attempting to achieve these aims and objectives is important.

REFERRAL DATA

Some form of referral data will be available for all but the most fleeting of client encounters, and the interviewer should ensure that she has access to all such information. All referral information shares two key characteristics. First, such information is collected in a biased way – it represents what some other party has discovered about the client's experiences and difficulties, and it is unlikely that such discoveries represent a total or accurate record. The opinion of experts is subject to systematic distortion by time, personality, and the expert's own interviewing style (Thompson, 1984a; Newell, 1992). One near exception to this is the self-referral letter. Whilst there is no reason to suppose that the report of the client herself will necessarily be more accurate than that of some third party, and whilst it also should, therefore, be treated with caution, it is, nevertheless, clear that the self-referral letter offers additional important information by (a) giving the interviewer an insight into the client's *feelings* about the difficulties in a way no third party could, and (b) giving potentially accurate information about the impact of the difficulties on the client's life. Such information is less likely to be present in a professional referral, I suggest, because of the gap between professional and client concerns discussed in the previous chapter (Dillon, 1990). Second, referral information is possibly mixed with irrelevant opinion about the client. Remarks made by professionals about unpopular, demanding clients are likely to be very different from those made about popular, compliant ones.

These difficulties of biased information collection and opinionated information transmission have led some interviewers to omit reading of referral data until after the interview has occurred, in an effort to reduce the bias brought to the interview situation. Although this is a laudable aim, it is not recommended. The interviewer cannot afford to approach the interview situation with less than the maximum opportunity to amass information beforehand. It gives the client an impression of unpreparedness on the part of the interviewer, which may lessen both the client's estimation of clinician competence and of the clinician's respect for her. These perceptions are, it should be noted, perfectly accurate. The poorly prepared interviewer offers quite direct evidence to the client of lack of competence and respect. These qualities are associated with poor client compliance. One way of dealing with this issue is to share the agenda with the client by explaining why the referral information has not been read.

It is suggested, however, that the information available from referral sources *may* offer a valuable orientation to the interview. Indeed, any biases we pick up in the referral information may themselves orientate us towards possible difficulties with the interview ahead. For instance, the client who has had difficulties in making earlier clinicians understand her needs may, quite reasonably, have a number of negative views about the consultation procedure and the role of experts in general. These difficulties of bias and opinion may be lessened by offering clients the opportunity to present a rich account of their own views of the problem. In this context, biases in the referral document should assume less salience.

RESOURCES

Here, the interviewer may be able to make, from the referral data, reasonable assumptions about what kind of human or other resources may be required. In particular, the interviewer should note whether the interviewee is *likely* to present problems which tax her current level of therapeutic skill towards the limit of what seems reasonable. Does it appear that the client's difficulty is such that the nurse will require specialized consultations or supervision from other health care professionals? Even if the nurse is familiar with the problems the client brings to the interview, the role in which the nurse finds herself may be unfamiliar. For example, only advice to other professionals, or the offering of supervision of their interventions with the client, may be required. Is the interviewer clear about how such needs will be met? More practically, if the client is taken into treatment, will travelling be necessary for client or nurse? Will co-therapists living near the client be required? Is it likely that special equipment will be needed to help the nurse and client work together?

RECORDS

The competent interviewer is aware of the need for appropriate record-keeping of all but the most brief and trivial encounter with a client, and ensures before the interview that the necessary papers, score sheets, recording devices are available and to hand. This also serves as a reminder to the clinician to check issues regarding records with the client. Is a system of open record-keeping practised? What expectations or rights does the client have or desire with regard to confidentiality? Is permission needed for some unusual monitoring procedure (e.g. audio or video recording)? The nurse may also feel that some further recording by the client (such as diary keeping) may be required after the end of the session, and again should have the necessary paperwork ready.

POSSIBLE OUTCOMES

From your knowledge of other interviews, and of clients who *appear*, from the referral data, to have similar difficulties, consider what the possible likely outcomes are from the first interview. Will there be a wait before treatment? What will you do if treatment is not appropriate, either at this time or in this setting? Supposing the client does not agree to intervention by you? A brief examination of these possibilities will serve to help focus the clinician's mind on practical aspects of the task ahead, and are particularly useful in focussing on those aspects of the interview concerned with closure, another key aspect of the consultation process.

SETTING

It is helpful to the interviewer to consider what kind of setting the interview is taking place in, and, again, to attempt to tailor the interview conditions so as to optimize the chance of a successful encounter with the client. Extraneous noise not only distracts, and if especially intrusive, raises stress levels, but should also be avoided so as to avoid the impression of lack of privacy. Physical surroundings are rarely ideal, and so this counsel of excellence cannot always be adhered to. In this case, *share the problem with the client* once the interview has begun. In extreme situations, the interview may need to be rescheduled or resited.

Physical aspects of the surroundings other than noise and lack of privacy may also be problematic. It is often suggested, for example, that chairs of different heights, or in certain orientations are best avoided. Although there is little empirical work relating to arrangement of chairs during interviews, Sommer (1959) found that people interacting socially preferred chairs to be placed at an angle to each other, rather than directly opposite. An ideal distance between participants will be around three to four feet, reflecting something between intimate and casual/personal distance (Argyle, 1969), and allowing the possibility of touch. Clearly, in a multiuser clinic room it will often be impossible to conform to such standards. Equally, an interview conducted at the client's bedside will very likely break all these guidelines for effective communication. Prior to interview, the interviewer needs to be aware of these issues, so that they can be discussed with the client.

As a final aspect of setting, the clinician should consider who is likely to be present. If the client is being interviewed in conjunction with others (for example family members or supportive friends), how will their contribution to the proceedings be handled? In general, the interviewer can opt for a structured approach, in which the client is the main contributor, and others are not asked for comments until the end of the interview, or may run the interview as essentially a group experience, in which all participants contribute throughout.

Although this distinction is, in a sense, artificial, and should, in any case, be negotiated with the client, interviews with a number of people will resemble one or other of the extremes noted here. Both have drawbacks. The structured interview is problematic because participants other than the client may have valuable contributions based on client remarks at any stage of the interview, which they may forget if they are restricted by having to save their remarks until some later stage. By contrast, the 'group interview' approach may result in information overload for the interviewer, who may be involved in a struggle to process a series of quite different elements form the different sources.

Prior to the interview, however, the interviewer has the opportunity to decide on what format she will employ, and should, at that stage, have due regard to her own level of expertise in dealing with the competing demands of the two interviews. The difficulties of both styles may then be shared with the client, in the hope of arriving at a way of proceeding which maximizes the potential for information transfer.

A special example of interviewing more than one person is the couple interview, where both partners identify themselves as the clients, as in marital therapy, sex therapy and certain other situations (e.g. bereavement counselling). Aspects of the group interview are returned to in Chapter 5.

As an aid to memory, consider the mnemonic TARPS, which is derived from the above considerations, and refers to the skilled interviewer's need, before each interview, to plan and check the following points:

(T)IMING

Check how much time there is for the interview and be punctual.
Plan how much can be achieved within the time constraints. How many clients constitute a reasonable caseload?

(A)IMS AND OBJECTIVES

Check that you have considered general aims and objectives which are true for all interviews of this kind (e.g. admission, intervention, discharge interview).
Plan specific aims and objective for *this* interview, with *this* client.

(R)EFERRAL DATA

Check that this information has been read analytically and sympathetically, and remembered.
Plan on the basis of any unusual elements of the referral information whether these will affect the current interview or whether they need raising with the client.

(R)ESOURCES

Plan what special resources will be required.
Check that they are available.

(R)ECORDS

Check that appropriate aids to record-keeping are accessible.
Plan discussion with the client of any issues regarding records, including permission-seeking.

(P)OSSIBLE OUTCOMES

Check that you have considered these.
Plan tentatively what tactics you will use in each eventuality.

(S)ETTING

Check that physical aspects of the setting conform to the optimum possible for effective communication.
Plan how you will deal with divergences from this optimum level.
Check who will be present.
Plan how to deal with groups.

THE INTERVIEW ITSELF – ENGAGING WITH THE CLIENT

We have already seen how important the initial stages of an interview are, for both client and clinician. We will now examine how the interviewer can employ simple opening tactics to optimize the impact of the opening on the interviewing relationship. Most of these are familiar to us from everyday use, but, as Maguire (1979) noted, seem absent from clinical interviews, and may even have been 'unlearnt' by clinicians through a process of modelling based on the performance of higher status clinicians who are, however, ineffective interviewers.

Greeting

Here, the interviewer seeks to reduce potential client anxiety by orienting the client to the material to follow. First, the interviewer establishes the client's name. Although this is a simple issue of respect, in a busy clinic, there is also a practical issue, in that it is important to ascertain that the correct client is being interviewed.

Next, the interviewer introduces herself by name, and also states her role, interviewer behaviours which are by no means universal (Maguire & Rutter, 1976). This process may be longer than it at first seems. It is unlikely that such distinctions as 'sister', 'staff nurse', 'student nurse', and so on, will provide clients with much information. Role statement in interviews should, therefore, be non-institutional and be sufficiently accurate to leave the client in absolutely no doubt as to what the interviewer can generally be expected to do, both with the client herself and with clients generally. It should, therefore, describe briefly but accurately, in lay terms, what the clinician does or tries to do. Accordingly:

> 'In my work, I try, through talking to people about events, thoughts and feelings, to help them come to terms with how they feel when someone close to them has died.'

might be an adequate general statement by a grief counsellor, whereas:

> 'I am the grief counsellor attached to this hospital'

or:

> 'I discuss people's feelings with them'

are both inadequate, since the first is too institutional and the second too vague, and both are uninformative.

It is worth taking time to explain role early in the interview. As well as setting the client at ease by decreasing uncertainty, this tactic alerts the client to the type of information likely to be required and gives her the opportunity to voice any disquiet about the nature of the consultation. Not all clinicians will practise the same open agenda commended to readers of this book, and so the client may have expectations of the interview which diverge widely from what is likely to be on offer. For example, the client referred by her doctor to a pain clinic may assume that this is with a view to offering a new medication or operation, but the pain clinic may aim to offer a range of tactics involving problem-solving training from a behaviour therapist, massage from a physiotherapist, aromatherapy from an aromatherapist or self-hypnosis from a hypnotherapist. The point at issue is that the client is aware from an early stage in the interview what your likely intentions are, based on your therapeutic background and skills. This issue is, therefore, introduced for negotiation, in a general way, early in the consultation.

As part of the general orientation process, the interviewer can also, by mention of the referral agent and process, seek to set the consultation into context for the client. There are three points to this tactic. The interviewer attempts to make links with previous consultations so as to stress the importance of the current consultation, with the hope of increasing the likelihood that the client will offer the best information available. Second, it is possible that reference to earlier interviews might enhance client information giving by reminding them of issues still on their personal agenda, and helping them to link these to what happens during the current consultation. Certainly, there is considerable evidence in the educational literature that this kind of linking is helpful to learning and memory, since people are more likely to recall information which is meaningful to them (Wittrock, 1989). Finally, the interviewer puts the referring agent and the referral process onto the agenda, so that the client may, if necessary, express dissatisfaction, or seek to address issues which, in her view, were insufficiently covered during interviews with others. One particular link which may be important for the client is to note any particular differences between the current interview and previous experiences the client may have had.

Scene-setting

It is worth recognizing with the client any unusual aspects of the setting of the current interview. It may, for example, be the client's first experience of attending the hospital, clinic or other facility. Acknowledging this, or finding out from the client, is a useful way of expressing to the client, from the outset, that her experience is valued. If others are present (either with the client, or with the interviewer), this again should be recognized and the rationale for their presence explored. In the case of the clinician, permission for the presence of others, whether colleagues or students, should always be sought. It should not, however, be taken for granted that friends or relatives present with the client are necessarily there with her consent. Whether this is so should also be tactfully probed at this stage.

Agenda-setting: 1 – Time

Stating how long the interview is likely to last is helpful because it enables the client to order her thoughts and prioritize what she wants to discuss. Lessening uncertainty in this way also reduces anxiety. Finally, the client is orientated to the likely demands to be made upon her attention.

Agenda-setting: 2 – Content

How far the agenda can be negotiated, with regard to content, will depend upon the type of interview, the role of the clinician, and the individual client. What is important is that the offer of negotiation is made. The more involved the client is in the interview process, the better the quality of the information she offers will be. Furthermore, when intervention is made, there is greater likelihood that the client will adhere to any treatment instructions which are offered, since the client will feel 'ownership' of the intervention process (Thompson, 1984a).

In general, therefore, the interviewer should state her interpretation of how the interview is likely to proceed, in terms of likely content and the order in which that content will be introduced, setting that content into the context of the aims and objectives the clinician has for the interview. This can lead naturally to inquiry about the client's own goals from the interview, and the clinician can then examine with the client how far their goals are compatible and negotiate how to proceed. Once again, the overall aim of this tactic is to reduce client uncertainty and increase the likelihood of the client making the best possible use of her attention, and, ultimately, the time set aside for the interview (Ley, 1982). Clearly it is possible that no room for negotiation may exist, because the goals of interviewer and client are so at variance. This will be particularly so with the client who has come for treatment under some form of coercion. Nevertheless, it is important that even this inability to negotiate forms part of the agenda. Interactions with reluctant clients are examined in greater detail in Chapter 5.

Early negotiation

It should now be apparent that the opening of any interview offers the clinician a chance to set the scene for the therapeutic relationship, and also to give the client an experience, in miniature, of what interacting with her will be like in the future. Returning to the idea of 'first impressions', the interviewer aims to capitalize on our tendency to emphasize such impressions, by demonstrating to the client the likelihood that engaging in the interview will be likely to be a useful activity. This the interviewer does by demonstrating relevant expertise (Korsch *et al.*, 1968) and concern for the client's individuality and situation. The demonstration of relevant expertise is known to be an excellent predictor of client behaviour and confidence in the clinician, unlike general symbols of power and expertise (white coats, badges, stethoscopes). With regard to concern for the client, the nurse aims to demonstrate that, even when quite didactic interactions occur, there is always the possibility of negotiation with her. Thus, from the first interview, the client should be made to feel involved in the therapeutic process, and have knowledge both that treatment will be likely to depend in large measure on her own behaviour and that, in consequence, she also has rights within the therapeutic liaison.

At the beginning of the interview, these rights include the right to know all of the above information regarding what will occur. In addition, the client should be made aware of the likely outcomes of the interview in practical terms. For example, is it likely that explanation about possible interventions will be forthcoming, or is the interview purely for assessment purposes? Will the interviewer be involved with the client again in the future, or will intervention be left to some other clinician? What say will the client have in the process of treatment? These are *general* statements of interviewer intent and related client expectation. At the beginning of an interview, particularly at the beginning of a therapeutic relationship, they can be no more, and it is the interviewer's responsibility to make this clear, and to ensure that neither she nor the client are unduly constrained by such statements.

We now have a *minimum* set of criteria for beginning a successful interview with a client. Here, the mnemonic ILSSE may offer some help in remembering and organizing these criteria:

(I)NTRODUCTIONS

Who are you, who am I, what I do.

(L)INKS

Links with previous experiences and the referring agent.

(S)ETTING THE SCENE

Where we are, who is present, why.

(S)ETTING THE AGENDA

Timing, what will happen, state aims, elicit aims.

(E)ARLY NEGOTIATIONS

Relevant expertise, concern, likely outcomes and expectations, client roles and rights.

CASE MATERIAL

The following two case examples aim to illustrate, from two different nursing contexts, coping with beginning interviews.

Case example 1

Inter: Good Morning . . . David Forster?

Client: That's right.

Inter: Hello, Mr Forster. Please have seat. What I'd like to do, if I can, is to start by explaining a bit about who I am and how *I* see our interview going. I also hope you will be able to tell me later what your own expectations are in coming here. Does that sound OK?

Client: Yes, that's fine.

Inter: Well, first of all, I'm Susan Williams, and my job here at the clinic is to try and help people cope with their difficulties by learning specific psychological techniques, rather than by using medication. I am a trained nurse, with additional training in using these methods, and I especially work with problems such as fears and phobias. Is this anything like what you were expecting?

Susan's description of her role is highly specific, and she deliberately uses such phrases as 'try and help' and 'cope with their difficulties', rather than setting up false expectations about easy outcomes. She describes herself as a nurse only after *this, and does so only to emphasise her later training which is specific to her current role. Finally, she avoids referring to the client's difficulty – although she has some idea of it from the referral letter, but still cues the client to her experience in dealing with such difficulties, before eliciting the client's expectations.*

Client: Yes, pretty much. I told my doctor I wasn't interested in pills, and she said this place might be able to help. Actually, I think it's sort of a phobia I've got!

Inter: Yes, your doctor's letter, which I read earlier, in preparation for our meeting, says something of the kind, and that's the sort of thing I hope to go into with you as our conversation continues. Let me just say a few more words about how that might go.

Susan offers an initial orientation to the material to follow, and also demonstrates appropriate pre-interview behaviour to the client. She also swops the word 'interview' for the less formal 'conversation'.

Client: Right-o.

Inter: Over the next half hour, I hope to get a clear picture from you of the difficulties you are facing, and to decide in my own mind whether the methods I use will be helpful. I understand you've had to wait some weeks for this appointment, so I hope it will be worthwhile for you, and that you yourself will feel free to discuss with me what you hope to get out of our meeting. In fact, that's actually the first thing I'll be asking you.

Susan clearly states her timescale and aim for the interview, and implicitly prepares the client for the role of information-giver. She also shows concern for the client by referring to waiting time, and her hopes for a satisfactory outcome, whilst making an early offer of openness in the agenda, which the client then takes up.

Client: Thank you. Actually, my main concern is whether I'll be able to get back to work. At the moment, I've been off sick for ten weeks, and my boss is starting to ask questions! So I was hoping to get some answers today about what's the matter with me. Also, how long it will take to get over it. I've read this book about phobias by Doctor Smart (shows book) and haven't had much luck. Have you seen it?

Inter: Yes, I have read Dr Smart's book. I'm sorry you've not had much luck with it, but I'm glad to hear you've been 'having a go', so to speak. I'll ask you about what you've been doing with the book a bit later on. For now, let me say first of all that we're right at the beginning of the interview, and so I can't guarantee to have an absolute answer to your questions by the end of it. Still, I will certainly keep in mind the pressure you're under from the boss, and, hopefully, by the time we've talked a bit I'll be able to work towards the answers you're after. At the very least, I should be able to offer you some general advice in this session, and certainly be able to tell you whether the treatments I offer will help. If they can, I'll then be in a position to make an estimate of how successful treatment is likely to be, and also tell you about what's involved, what you'd be expected to do, and how long it will all take. I'd also ask you if you wanted to go ahead, having heard about it. At the moment, if treatment was suitable, I'd see us working together through to the end of, er, you know, the course of treatment.

Susan is familiar with the self-help book, but avoids discussion at this stage. She does, however, again demonstrate concern for the client, and also reinforces his attempt at self-help, before returning to the issue of agenda-setting and negotiation. She is careful to avoid making promises she cannot keep (since she does not know how the interview will turn out) but does make those assurances she can (those to do with the structure of the interview) and finishes her introductory remarks regarding what the client can expect from her.

Client: So I'd see you in future, then?

Inter: Yes, if we both agreed to go on with treatment, and you had no strong objection to our working together. Otherwise we might need to talk about a change.

Susan again emphasizes the negotiated, collaborative nature of treatment.

Client: I see. No, that's fine.

Inter: Thank you. Well, are there any other things you want to ask about the way the interview will go, before we get into it?

Client: No, I understand you need to find out some things before you can say much else about the problem (Smiles).

Inter: (Smiles) That's right. Now I wonder if I could begin by asking . . .

In the above example, Susan performs very well, dealing with a cooperative client who has quite clear expectations, it seems, about what to expect. Susan needs only to attend carefully to her own agenda and fit this to the client's few uncertainties. In the following example, however, Jean, a practice nurse, has to be slightly more directive in beginning an interview with a client about her leg ulcers.

Case example 2

Inter: Good afternoon. Mrs Sims, is it?

Client: That's it, love.

Inter: Thank you for coming, Mrs Sims. Do sit down. I'm hoping to start off by explaining why Dr Davies asked you to come along today, and also who I am, and what I do here at the health centre. I expect you also have your own ideas about why you are here, and I hope we can talk about those, too. Is that OK?

Client: Yes.

Inter: Well, my name is Jean Smith, I'm one of the nurses here, and I'm usually asked to talk to people and advise them on how to cope with health problems. I particularly look at how people are managing with practical things like taking medicine, dressings, getting about and so on.

So far, so good. Even if the 'and so on' is a little vague, it puts the interview into the appropriate conversational style. Jean's opening follows the approach used by Susan very closely. But . . .

Client: Yes, well, the main thing for me is getting my prescriptions. My daughter used to get them for me, but she hardly ever has time since she started work again. Also, getting out to the shops is very difficult, and general housework, too. Oh, and would you be able to help me to claim benefit?

For Jean, the problem is that she must choose how to continue with her agenda – setting the scene and so on – whilst avoiding alienating the client by appearing to ignore her legitimate concerns. This is particularly difficult, since Jean herself cued the client with her mention of getting about. The client, however, may well want to talk in much more general terms – for example about her relationship with her daughter – and has also raised a whole series of concerns at a very early stage in the interview.

Inter: This does sound difficult, and is part of what I was thinking about when I mentioned difficulty getting about. I hope we can return to it later. You also started to mention some other issues, like about your benefit, which I have only general knowledge about. I would still welcome discussing them with you, though, because I might at least be able to put you in touch with someone with more specialist knowledge. For the moment, let me just mention that we have about half an hour to talk, and during this time I hope we can discuss what the difficulties with your leg ulcers are (since that's the chief reason Dr Davies has asked you to see me), but also talk about what impact these difficulties have had on your life more generally. I'll also need, with your permission, to take a look at your legs. I myself can probably give you some quite specific advice on how to cope with the ulcers in a practical sense, and, as I said, possibly discuss with you the possibility of seeing someone else about other issues, like the benefit. Does that sound like a reasonable way to proceed?

Jean probably deals with this in the best way available. She starts by acknowledging the validity of the client's comments, and also validates their being stated at this time (by linking them to her own remarks). She then ties them to her own agenda item of discussing likely outcomes, and steers the conversation back to general introductory remarks, whilst assuring the client that her concerns will be dealt with. However, Jean must be sure that she does, in reality, return to these concerns, otherwise the client will take away the impression that they are not of interest to Jean. In some sense, if Jean does not return to the issues raised by the client, this impression is, indeed, true!

Client: Yes, that's all right. You ask away.

Inter: Thank you. I hope that you will ask me questions as we go along, too. It's very important that we both understand each other as much as possible.

Jean notices the slightly passive role suggested by the client's last utterance (and possibly caused in part by Jean's redirection of the conversation), and so emphasizes the need for a collaborative venture.

A NOTE ABOUT SMALL TALK

Some interviewers find that trivial social conversation (about the weather, and so on) is helpful in reducing client anxiety at the beginning of the interview, particularly at a first meeting. No doubt there are good reasons for this, in terms of showing the human face of the interviewer and offering the client safe, familiar conversational topics. However, in the absence of clear evidence for the effectiveness of this tactic, it is recommended that the sensitive interviewer uses it judiciously. The client may well either have been waiting a long time for the appointment, or have invested a great deal in its possible outcome. In either case, it is difficult to see how prolonging the agony before actually beginning to discuss sensitive or difficult topics helps to reduce anxiety. From the cognitive-behavioural perspective, this looks rather like an avoidance on the part of both client and interviewer, and is, perhaps, best dispensed with, both in view of what we know about client preference for focussed interviewing (Ley, 1977), and because of the message we will wish to send to clients that talking about sensitive issues is acceptable and safe for both client and interviewer. Moreover, cognitive-behaviourists in particular, but also interviewers from other therapeutic orientations, will want to keep the interview situation reserved for those aspects of communication which are the business of that interview. In other words, they will view irrelevant material as distracting the client and sending conflicting cues about the need to attend to what is being said by both participants. As a rule, they will want to discuss only highly focal topics within the interview room, and thus maximize the specificity of that situation for the client and, hopefully, capitalize on specific context-dependent recall (Anderson & Bower, 1973).

Social chit-chat is best confined, at least in the more formal interviewing situation, to the walk between collecting the client from the waiting area and arriving in the interviewing room, where business begins, demarcating the interview room as an area where specific types of communication take place. It is natural and appropriate to want to set the client at ease at the beginning of an interview, and it would be a mistake to train the humanity out of interviewers (Maguire, 1979). Nevertheless, it is suggested that, unless there is good evidence that the 'small talk gambit' is actually effective in reducing client anxiety in *clinical* situations, other tactics are used — essentially those which have been outlined and recommended during this chapter.

EXERCISES

1 Read the second interview again. The main alternative to the tactic adopted by Jean would be to follow the client's cues and embark on a discussion of each of the client concerns raised by Mrs Sims. It is often valid and important to do so.

Imagine how the interview might have gone if Jean had adopted this tactic now. Focus in particular on:

Time available.
Orientation of the client.
Jean's own expertise.
Jean's own aims.

2 Decide how you would apply the opening structure offered in this chapter to your own clinical practice. Not all interviews are clinic-based, and not all are this formal. For example, how would the admitting nurse approach the newly-admitted client? How would the health visitor appropriately commence an interview on visiting a mother at home? Write an aide-memoire to enable you to employ the adapted structure.

3 The TARPS and ILSSE formats represent a series of objectives for use at the beginning of interviews. Consider what your own objectives might be, and how these relate to TARPS and ILSSE.

FURTHER READING

Ley, P. (1977) Psychological studies of doctor-patient communication. *In* S. Rachman (ed.) *Contributions to Medical Psychology*. Oxford. Pergamon Press.
Maguire, P. (1979) Teaching essential interviewing skills to medical students. *In* D.J.Oborne, M.M.Gruneberg & J.R.Eiser (eds) *Research in Psychology and Medicine*, Vol. II. London. Academic Press.

3   Learning from interviews

In the previous chapter, we examined a structure for beginning interviews, and offered exercises which sought to help you apply this structure to your own interviews. From now on, the exercises will increasingly invite you to begin conducting real interviews, in order to maximize your learning and examine for yourself the effect of the strategies which have been suggested. As part of this process, you will need some way of assessing your developing abilities as your interviewing progresses. So, this chapter sets out to provide exactly those strategies needed for reviewing your attempts at achieving excellence in interviewing. To this end we shall look at both a series of practical approaches to examining our interviewing and a general conceptual context into which those techniques fit, through the notion of reflecting about interviewing, which is commended to the reader as a method of examining interviewing practice. Practical aspects of the need for record-keeping will be examined at the close of the chapter, within the context of reflection about practice, but also since record-keeping should, logically, begin with the first encounter, however brief.

LEARNING FROM INTERVIEWS BY REFLECTION

A number of interviewing situations offer clinicians the opportunity to gain from direct feedback on their interviewing performance. Certainly, many educational settings offer this possibility, using intensive video work to allow the clinician to examine her developing performance, often immediately after it has occurred, with the help of a teacher or other colleague. This kind of video review is also increasingly available for the trained nurse in mental health settings, particularly in organizations which take a psychotherapeutic approach to client care. It is, however, a rare occurrence in nursing as a whole. Although video is an extremely powerful aid to learning, and to the reflective process more generally, it is not without serious drawbacks. As we have noted, video facilities are not available in all settings. In particular, the general nurse who has completed training and is now experiencing early difficulties associated with conducting unsupervised or minimally supervised nursing assessments is unlikely to have access to such facilities. Furthermore, even where video facilities are available, time constraints will often rule out their use, and not all clients will consent to participate. Both these issues suggest that, where video recording does occur, it is unlikely to be with a representative sample of either interview situations or clients – only those interviews where time is plentiful and which involve cooperative clients being likely to be available for examination. This is unfortunate, since the nurse will want access to a cross-section of interviews, so as to permit examination of both strengths and weaknesses. It is these drawbacks which lead to the consideration of reflection on practice as the most important readily accessible tool the clinician can use in attempting to learn from interviews.

Reflection is an ability to examine one's own actions, thoughts and feelings, and, by reviewing a 'repertoire of clinical experience and knowledge' (Saylor, 1990), to modify professional practice in the face of complex, constantly changing situations. It is regarded by many authors as a key issue in the development of professional knowledge and judgement, whether in the field of research, teaching or clinical practice, and is described by Schon (1983) as the creative process whereby novel solutions are found to professional problems at work. Numerous writers (e.g. Dewing, 1990) have outlined methods of facilitating reflection by the use of diaries, group discussion and support, and relaxation techniques. Of these, the reflective journal remains the most widely advocated tool for promoting reflection on practice.

Although a distinction is made between reflection-in-practice, which occurs during the performance of a particular act, and reflection-on-practice, which involves later examination of it, both are essentially reconstructions of the experiences to-be-reflected-upon, through recall of events, thoughts and feelings. In an examination of reflection in nursing practice, from which some of the material in the early part of this chapter is drawn (Newell, 1992), I have argued that such recall is subject to systematic bias because of setting, manner of presentation of information, mood and anxiety level. Nevertheless, it is also the case that more reliable but equally practical methods of examining one's professional experiences are not currently available. Therefore, despite this fallibility, reflection represents the clinician's best option, particularly since it has the great advantage of potentially being a continuous process which can be adopted by the developing interviewer in any situation, without recourse to special equipment. The shortcomings of reflection, should, however, be briefly stated, since they provide the rationale for many of the specific tactics I shall suggest to you.

Anderson & Bower (1973) have described a good deal of evidence that recall of information is related to variables associated with the acquisition of memories. These may be divided into effects of context – the surroundings in which memories are acquired – and effects of state – the internal state of the person acquiring such memories. In both cases, it is a reliable finding that the more state and context differ between the situation when information was acquired and that in which it is remembered, the less accurate the memory is likely to be. As well as being important for reflection, this finding also has implications for transmitting information to the client, and we will visit it again when we discuss educating and advising. Interviewers and clients are equally at risk from these sources of inaccuracy.

As well as being an element in an individual's internal state, anxiety level has another effect on accuracy of recollection. Baddeley (1983) notes that memory is likely to be improved by modest levels of arousal, but impaired as levels continue to rise. Interviews can be a time of anxiety for interviewers (especially novice interviewers), as well as for clients, and this may cause difficulty in recalling the events. Most particularly, problematic elements of interviews may give rise to greater increase in anxiety, with increased impairment of recall.

This anxiety may also lead to avoidance of both stressful interviews and stressful components of interviews. In this case, difficult material, reflection on which may lead to interviewing excellence, is simply unavailable to the interviewer, leading to the mistaken impression that there are no difficulties which need to be addressed, an inappropriate tactic we mentioned when discussing problems with interviewing in Chapter 1. Reflection relies on our attempting to enter those situations which cause anxiety, and remaining open to as many anxiety-provoking elements of the situation as possible. Sundeen *et al.* (1989) discuss avoidance tactics as attempts to preserve the integrity of the self by limiting our awareness of experiences, in the face of threats to self-esteem. They suggest that such tactics limit potential for change and growth in the individual, whilst for interviewing, it is clear that they greatly reduce the opportunity for practice, the attempting of novel tactics and reflection about such innovations in interviewing technique.

So far, we have discussed how experiences fail to form part of our memories, owing to constraints operating on the memory task and individual variations during the time at which memories are acquired. By contrast, information may be available in memory, but be incapable of retrieval, chiefly because of anxiety associated with the information to be retrieved. In this context, cognitive-behaviourists argue that such memories are avoided because avoidance is rewarding to the interviewer. The reward is escape from experiencing the unpleasant feelings of anxiety associated with such memories, and the long-term consequence is that the memories become less and less well recalled, since inability to retrieve them is continually rewarded in the way I have described. In view of this, it is likely that interviewers will tend to recall only the least threatening information. This possibility, coupled with the suggestion above that anxiety-provoking situations are less likely to be accurately stored in memory in the first place, is again problematic, since it may give rise, during reflection (or during supervision from a colleague) to an account of the interview process which is characterized by bland and unthreatening recollections. The concomitant danger of this is that there will be little for the interviewer to learn from a process of reflection in which everything seems to go right!

IMPROVING YOUR REFLECTIVE ABILITY

Aids to memory

Given the limitations examined above, it is clear that the practitioner intending to use reflection to enhance interviewing skills faces numerous difficulties.

Nevertheless, I have also stressed the necessity of reflection, given the unavailability of other options in the refinement of clinical practice. Therefore, attempting reflection in a systematic way which avoids as many as possible of the potential difficulties I have described is of paramount importance.

The reflective diary has already been mentioned, and may form the core of your reflective tactics. Most researchers agree that journals should contain details of the event being examined, together with the thoughts and feelings the event gives rise to. For the purpose of reflecting about interviewing, we shall be working with the 'where, when, what, who with, how long' approach described by Richards & MacDonald (1990). This approach has been examined and advocated by numerous writers in the cognitive-behavioural tradition, notably Marks (1986), and is also closely related to numerous systematic recording schedules introduced in nursing and medicine. It is allied to the three systems model of Lang (1971), which describes the interaction between the behavioural, physical and cognitive elements of any given situation. Both the specific assessment strategies and the three systems model will be discussed in some detail in the following two chapters, since they also form the model of assessment which we will follow when we examine information gathering and handling. Thus, you will be able to benefit from continuity in terms of the tactics you use during interviews and those you use to enhance your reflection about them. For the present, however, to introduce you to the approach, the following format (Figure 3.1) is suggested as a diary record for your interviewing during both the exercises associated with this book and your efforts at enhancing interviewing during your

DATE	EVENT	WHAT HAPPENED (where, who with, who said what)	THOUGHTS AT THE TIME	ACTION TO BE TAKEN

Notes:
EVENT – e.g. assessment interview, home visit, discharge
THOUGHTS – as detailed as possible – include feeling states
ACTION – to include reflections nowand ideas for action during future events and ideas on further reflections

Figure 3.1 Diary recording sheet

clinical practice more generally. Perhaps more important, however, than the use of any particular schedule of recording is the need for *some* schedule, so that the practitioner has the best possible chance of being able to examine important aspects of critical events in clinical practice. If we simply recall such information at a later date, there is great likelihood of the schematized reconstruction suggested earlier.

To help with accurate recall of events, record these *as near the time of the event as possible*. This will decrease the interference with memory likely to occur when further events intervene. Attempting to diminish the effects of context and state dependency is also important, and so recording should also take place in an environment as similar as possible to that in which the interview took place (in the same room, if possible). Even if it is not possible to spend much time in reflection so soon after a critical event has occurred, any immediate recording will be helpful later in providing cues to memory which reduce the burden of the memory task by making it a recognition exercise, where the practitioner recognizes events, thoughts and feelings by reference to her writings from the time of the event itself. Recognition memory tasks are acknowledged to be far easier than recall in the absences of cues. Group discussion may serve the same function, offering recall cues from the remarks of others on the interview which has occurred.

As well as writing full journal reports of therapeutic interactions, checklists can also be useful, since you can orient yourself to particular issues you hope to address beforehand and simply note the occurrence of such issues on either a mental or actual checklist. In so doing, you may decide deliberately to narrow the focus of what you will attempt to observe and reflect about, perhaps concentrating on one aspect of your verbal or non-verbal behaviour. Figure 3.2 gives a format for your use in checklists you can design yourself to examine specific aspects of your interviewing. The idea is to tick in the appropriate box each time you note a particular behaviour. In the example, the checklists attempts to examine whether the interviewer is asking too many closed questions, by looking both at interviewer behaviour and client behaviour.

Many of you will be familiar with open and closed questions and their supposed effect on the flow of information. In any event, these issues are

BEHAVIOUR	TICKS
Open question by nurse	✓✓✓
Closed question by nurse	✓✓✓✓✓
Yes/no answer by client	✓✓✓✓
Detailed, developed answer by client	

Figure 3.2 Sample checklist

discussed in Chapter 5 (see p. 70). For the moment, it is sufficient for you to note that the possibility exists of monitoring the occurrence of these types of question for yourself, and examining what effect they have during a particular interview. All interviewers have experienced, for example, the interview in which the client seems either to give very little information or to assume total control of the interview and swamp the interviewer with information. It is possible to use a checklist such as the one offered above to examine the relationship of these two response styles to types of questioning, and, indeed, to examine the effect of deliberately attempting to modify such responding by changing questioning style. Thus, after an interview in which the client's responses seem particularly vague, garrulous and unfocussed, you might decide to employ more closed questions, count these on the checklist, and observe their effect on the client's responses by counting the two types of response. Clearly, the use of this tactic should be negotiated with the client as far as possible. Once again, the use of this kind of negotiation about information handling is discussed in Chapter 5.

The use of checklists is not confined to the monitoring of behavioural aspects of interactions. We have already noted some of the defences we adopt in order to protect ourselves from feelings of inadequacy associated with difficulties in interviewing (for example, blaming clients for difficulties). When the occurrence of such thoughts is noted, a checklist can be constructed to examine their frequency in the same way we would a count the frequency of a piece of verbal or non-verbal behaviour during an interview. Indeed, monitoring of assumptions about clients could continue throughout all aspects of our clinical lives, to include writing up of notes, discussion with colleagues, writing of referral letters – even the reflective process itself!

As a final aspect of reducing reliance on memory, it is worth noting that all the suggestions offered for personal reflection apply equally to debriefing situations using supervisors or peers. These will need to occur as near as possible to the event to be recalled, in terms of both time and place, capitalizing on immediacy and upon state and context cues as far as possible, and here again the use of written aids to recall can be put to good use.

REDUCING ANXIETY

So far, we have discussed practical aids to recall, but it has also been noted that anxiety is a potent factor in interfering with memory, and therefore with our ability to reflect adequately about interviewing performance. For effective reflection, therefore, clinicians need effective anxiety management strategies. Although a supportive environment may be useful in reducing anxiety, specific interventions are often likely to be required. Clearly it is beyond the scope of this chapter to offer great detail about anxiety management, and several readable texts exist (see, for example, Bailey, 1985). Nevertheless, some reliable interventions can be suggested.

Of the responses to anxiety examined above, behavioural avoidance is probably of greatest importance to the clinician. If situations of interaction with clients are avoided completely, or if all but the most superficial are avoided, because of anxiety, then there is no possibility of increasing interpersonal effectiveness and interviewing skill. A first step is to identify such situations, and here, the reflective journal may help. Perhaps the clinician always avoids interactions with clients who have just returned from weekend leave, or from undergoing particular treatments, or always allocates clients with particular difficulties to other nurses. If you are a more experienced nurse, you may find yourself having to help less experienced interviewers to identify such weak spots. Indeed, as a clinical manager, it may even be such supervisory interviews with less experienced colleagues, or confrontative elements of such interviews, that *you* avoid.

Once such avoidances have been identified, the key issue seems to be gradual and repeated attempts to reinitiate such avoided behaviours, whilst journal-keeping continues, providing feedback on growing confidence. Although relaxation or meditative techniques may help facilitate this confrontation, it is the actual *exposure* to the anxiety-provoking situations which results in anxiety reduction (see Marks, 1987, for an extended academic account of the role of exposure in anxiety reduction, or Marks, 1980, for a brief, readable self-help guide which is equally useful for health professionals and their clients). Our natural tendency to cease to respond to anxiety-provoking stimuli in this way is a cornerstone of much cognitive-behavioural work, and is returned to several times throughout this book.

Where behavioural avoidance has not occurred, but the clinician has difficulty in remembering emotionally charged information from interviews, exposure in imagination can be helpful. This procedure is quite simply one of imagining past events as vividly as possible. It was used in early behaviour therapy interventions in preference to exposure in real life, and has latterly been found to be as effective, under certain conditions, as such real life exposure in evoking the anxiety associated with phobic avoidance (Richards, 1988). It is also used in the management of chronic pain, as the client seeks to gain mastery over the painful experiences. For the interviewer, the aim is to recall those painful or anxiety-provoking aspects of interviewing which are less likely to come into the memory than less problematic memories. The procedure can be undertaken alone or with a colleague, and is described in Figure 3.3. Spending about 10–15 minutes on the exercise is useful for recall of information. If the information is particularly emotionally charged (for the interviewer), then it can be useful to spend an extended amount of time repeatedly evoking the emotions, again using the phenomenon of repeated exposure to decrease associated anxiety. However, such anxiety will rarely reach such levels in interviews, and therefore the tactic of prolonged exposure will rarely be necessary. Although it is not dangerous, it can result in considerable levels of anxiety, and therefore, I recommend its use with the support of a supervisor who is knowledgeable about the process.

I have suggested that group discussion may aid the memory task, but it is also worth examining interviewing techniques in groups because of their usefulness in anxiety reduction. Clearly the support of peers can help us to discuss and examine problematic aspects of interviewing. Additionally, a regular group may

Sit comfortably in a quiet environment.

Close your eyes.

Begin to picture the interview you want to remember.

Describe what happened aloud, using the first person, present tense (e.g. Now I'm asking the client, 'tell me about your problem in general').

Imagine the scene using all five senses (sight, hearing, touch, taste and smell), and incorporate this into your description.

Also describe what you felt physically and your thoughts at the time of the interview.

When you are ready, open your eyes and examine the details you have recalled.

Figure 3.3 Exposure in imagination

set a series of agendas which examine specific areas of interviewing, and also address such general issues as anxiety management skills, modelling of appropriate disclosure about difficult interviews, problem-solving and supportive challenging about avoidances.

For the interviewer without access to the regular support of peers, a final tactic remains: the use of rehearsal. Here, the interviewer may practise tactics to be used in forthcoming interviews, and may focus on particular aspects of the interviewing task. Here the use of checklists can again be useful in orienting the interviewer, but in this context, the aim of rehearsal and checklist use is anxiety reduction, as the interviewer decides to focus on particular aspects of interviewing which have given rise to anxiety in the past.

RECORD-KEEPING

Throughout this chapter, we have examined the fallibility of memory and its interaction with the natural anxieties we all encounter in human interactions. So far, our discussion has focussed solely on the notion of reflection about interviewing practice, since I have suggested that it is primarily through the admittedly flawed process of reflection that we can begin to improve our interviewing through learning from experience. The fallibility of memory also has other consequences for the interviewer, however. Quite simply, without adequate record-keeping, information about the client, both in terms of the content and process of the interview, is lost. In consequence, later interviews are increased in their difficulty, since the interviewer is in an impoverished position with regard to making the best use of the information the client gives, by putting it in the context of relevant information from the past. This is true not only of forgotten content, where the interviewer lamely stumbles to remember what a client has previously said, but also with regard to forgotten process. If the interviewer has forgotten that a particular question or topic gave rise to difficulties in the interview on the last occasion interviewer and client met (for example, a silence, an episode of embarrassment for the client, apparent sadness), then she is unlikely to be able to deal with this effectively in the current interview if it occurs again.

Naturally, a good deal of the what we have looked at so far in terms of reflection bears upon these issues of forgotten content and process, since the reflective interviewer will be aware of both her tendency to overlook certain pieces of client information and certain aspects of client interactive style. However, there are also quite practical aspects to recording of client interactions. Information must be stored so that it can benefit the client by being available to other health care workers involved with her care, and so as to aid memory at some later date, when even the most conscientious interviewer may have forgotten a great deal about previous interactions. This immediately raises issues to do with both confidentiality and freedom of information which are beyond the scope of this book. In most settings, local policy directives will dictate what the inter-viewer must do to a large degree, but I again draw your attention to the practice of an open agenda with the client. If others must have access to your written records of an interaction, ensure that the client is aware of this. Negotiate with the client what will be recorded wherever possible. Negotiate also who will have access, where this is possible. Of course, there are some settings (e.g. forensic psychiatry) where the amount of negotiation is very small. Nevertheless, as in all other settings, the guideline is quite clear – as much openness and client autonomy as possible. Even where this is extremely restricted, the admission of this as part of the open agenda between interviewer and client will go a long way towards diminishing the impact of this upon the interview.

Marks (1986) has a useful handbook of how to deal with issues of recording in a clinical caseload, examined principally from a behavioural viewpoint, and most of my ideas about record-keeping come from my experiences of case management in behavioural settings. Most interviewers will not be working within such a framework, but many of the issues faced by behaviour therapists in terms of case management are common to all interviewers. The following are some very general guidelines about record-keeping.

Consider who will use the records. The content should be understandable to persons who have never met the client, yet brief enough to encourage the reader to read them carefully in their entirety. Thus, they should combine individual focus, precision and succinctness with completeness. Equally, the language should be understandable, and free from jargon. In particular, understanding of it should not rest upon understanding of a particular model of human experience, because records are descriptions of what occurred between you and the client, not your opinions. If you *must* describe the client's experience in terms of (say) Bandura's social learning theory, or Orem's self-care model, then the place to do this is during your formulation of the client's difficulties, which, although no doubt an

---

Client .... Nurse .... Date ....
Session Number ....

Topics – Sue talked about mother's funeral today. Repeated this several times to allow her to get accustomed to discussing it. I encouraged as much detail as possible. Her main recollection – the pace of the day – Sue organizing everything and everybody – no time for herself. Encouraged her to talk about what she would have spent time on if she had had it – mainly saying goodbye to mum and being sad by herself. This was first time she has talked about the funeral (10 years ago). She had decided this was what she wanted to discuss today, and so was reluctant about coming. Very tearful throughout, but able to say 'mum' repeatedly – previously impossible to do so.

After talking, still pretty low. Repeated discussion of funeral day once more, and Sue reported feeling calmer. Used this as opportunity to repeat rationale about anxiety reduction as result of repeated exposure.

Things at home are a bit better. Husband now accepts Sue needing to talk about mum.

Sue's homework – Think about day of mum's death for half an hour 3 times during the week. Get out holiday photos to bring here next time.

Plans for next session – Review homework. Look at photos with Sue for bulk of session. Negotiate homework.

Duration of this session ....
Total treatment duration ....
Date of next session ....

Figure 3.4 Record of a client interview

important aspect of record-keeping, is not part of an *interview* record. Incidentally, there are good reasons for *never* describing experiences in the interpretative way I have stated, both practical and theoretical, even in the formulation. If you share a theoretical orientation with whoever else reads the notes, theoretical descriptions are redundant; if you do not, they offer no help to the reader. More crucially, writing about people's experiences in theoretically-anchored terms represents a rehearsal of that way of examining their experience, and, therefore, a reinforcement of interaction with them according to that theoretical standpoint. This in turn takes the interviewer away from the *actual* experience of what the client is saying, and is, therefore, detrimental to the interviewing process. For this reason alone, records should also be as value-free as is possible.

Overwhelmingly, however, *records are kept for yourself*, as an aid in organizing the client's care and as an aid to management of a group of clients.

Here again, the use of succinct, jargon-free language which focuses on the individual will help, especially if you have to refer to notes again in the distant future. Client records should, therefore, provide a unique description of your interaction with each client, and should accurately reflect the content of each session. Beyond this, records should provide an opportunity for your comments on how your interventions with the client are progressing, and *planning for further sessions*. Finally, as an aid in *caseload planning*, records should contain details of the amount of time spent with the client, the number of sessions spent and estimated, and practical details such as the date and time of the current and next sessions. Figure 3.4 gives an example of a reasonable way of recording the events of an interaction, in this case with a grieving client. Note that the record does not attempt to be encyclopaedic. Such lengthy records are unlikely to be read again. Although they may serve a purpose in allowing the nurse to work out for herself aspects of a client's care, they are best destroyed after writing, and a more concise version recorded. The process of arriving at the precis in itself is potentially an aid to the thinking process, bringing clarity to the nurse's ideas about the client and the interview as part of the quest for the important features of the interaction, in the interests of brevity.

EXERCISES

1 During the previous chapter, we examined general aspects of first meetings. Draw up the following:

A general outline for recording the process and content of a first meeting with a client.
A general set of guidelines for reflecting about client interviews.
A checklist to examine your behaviour during a first interview with a client.

Remember that the examples given in this chapter are only to guide you. Your aids to reflection and record-keeping should be personal to your own clinical situation.

2 Most nurses work in situations where a good deal of the record-keeping is a matter of policy. Consider how far the suggestions given about record-keeping during interviewing are embodied in such policies, or how your current record-keeping might be changed to include them. The key issues are that the records:

are concise;
are jargon-free and value-free;
are personal to the client;
are complete and precise;
allow forward-planning for this client;
allow caseload-planning for a group of clients.

3 Conduct three initial interviews with clients according to your usual practice, but using the aids to reflection and recording you have devised. Consider the strengths and weaknesses both of your interviews and of the aids you have used.

FURTHER READING

Marks, I.M. (1980) *Living With Fear.* New York. McGraw-Hill.
Schon, D.A. (1987) *Educating the Reflective Practitioner: Towards a New Design for Teaching and Learning in the Professions.* San Francisco. Josey-Bass.

4   Elements of assessment interviewing

INTRODUCTION

In Chapter 2, we examined in some detail the way the skilled interviewer aims to set the scene for the material to follow, by orientating the client to her surroundings and to the process of the interview to follow. This is most often, in nursing, some kind of assessment interview, during which nurse and client are learning about each other. This chapter and Chapter 5 are both concerned with this increasing knowledge, examining both the content and process of the assessment interview. There is a great deal of material to be covered under this heading, and so I have dealt with more general issues regarding the process skills of information-gathering, negotiation and planning skills in Chapter 5, reserving the present chapter for an examination of the *structure, aims and components* of cognitive–behavioural (CB) interviewing. Thus, by the end of this chapter, you should have an awareness of the aims and rationale of CB assessment interviewing and of what sorts of information such assessment collects, along with skills in ordering the information collected.

THE NATURE OF ASSESSMENT

Although most descriptions of the nursing process draw a distinction between assessment, planning, implementation and evaluation, in practice the four processes can often be extremely closely linked. For example, it will be argued that the assessment phase of a nursing intervention is not only essential to evaluation, since it is during assessment that baseline information, without which evaluation is impossible, begins to be gathered, but is also an opportunity to initiate the client into the process of evaluation and stress its importance to intervention. Clearly, assessment can also form part of the implementation phase of treatment, both through the instigation of the nurse–client relationship, which can itself be therapeutic, and through the process of information-giving by the client, which can help to clarify problem definition and offer clues towards problem-solving. Nowhere, however, are the divisions less distinct than between assessment and planning. Whilst some writers wish to reserve the term 'assessment' purely for the process of information-gathering, others include a variety of activities as part of the assessment process. For example, Hunt & Marks-Maran (1980) include problem definition as part of a process of review of the information gained, whilst Richards & McDonald (1990) recognize the role of planning and evaluation in the assessment process. Other CB writers acknowledge also the inclusion of elements such as relationship-building, orientation to the therapeutic concepts underlying intervention and goal-setting within the assessment interview.

Perhaps it is best to reserve the expression 'assessment' for the activity of information gathering, whilst an 'assessment interview' may contain both this and the other related activities I have noted. Since this chapter and the next are about assessment *interviewing*, the broader range of activities will be discussed, although, clearly, it is possible to divide the activities into subsequent 'formulation interviews', 'planning interviews', and so on. However, the general sense of the literature seems to be that these are all highly related activities. For the purpose of these two chapters, I shall define assessment as the *process of defining, refining and negotiating a client's problems, within the context of her more general life history.* A related issue to the definition of assessment is the matter of timing. It is traditional to think of and describe assessment as an initial process, although more recent descriptions of the nursing process (e.g. Sundeen *et al.*, 1989) emphasize the continuing nature of assessment, with repeated reassessments of a client. Much of this reassessment, however, tends, in fact, to be evaluative in nature, in the sense that no new information about the client is introduced other than through the monitoring of changes in the client's status as a result of intervention. Reassessment, by contrast, takes into account the dynamic nature of the nurse–client relationship and the tendency for information about the client to continue to emerge in the context of growing trust between nurse and client. The conclusion to be drawn from this is that planning and implementation must also be constantly changing, to take account of the changing data. Practically speaking, however, such continuous assessment is logically impossible, since information would continue to emerge, and no plan of care could ever be drawn up or implemented which would take account of the continuing mass of data. Notable exceptions here would be those interventions which rely chiefly or solely on process (i.e. the therapeutic interaction of nurse and client itself) to effect change.

In reality, it seems that every interview consists of components of information-gathering, some of which are 'assessment', others 'evaluation'. Negotiations about intervention are made on the basis of both sorts of information-gathering and the associated activities described earlier. Nevertheless, most of assessment comes in the early stages of the nurse–client relationship, for reasons which are both practical and procedural. In the practical sense, the nurse seeks to obtain and the client seeks to give information in order to obtain changes in the client's difficulties. Procedurally, the transfer of information is part of the way in which the nurse and client find out about each other and begin their relationship: the nurse through eliciting information about the client; the client through seeing how the nurse deals with the information she has given.

Related to the idea of exchanging information in order to bring about changes in client problems is the issue of goal-setting, which again logically belongs in the early stages of the therapeutic relationship. Although there are some forms of counselling relationship which do not emphasize explicit goal-setting, these are becoming less common. Thus, whilst early descriptions of the helping relationship either do not discuss goals in any detail at all (Rogers, 1957) or see them as a late and minor stage of the counselling process (Newsome *et al.*, 1973), later, eclectic views of helping emphasize goals heavily (Egan, 1990) in a way which has always been true of cognitive and behavioural approaches. The role of goal-setting in assessment is another practical reason for suggesting that assessment is, in essence, a beginning in intervention, despite the continuing elements of it which crop up throughout treatment. Thus, this chapter deals with information acquisition skills in the context of a single interview, which examines the broad issues we have noted above. As ever, the issue is one of flexibility. Although most of the information-gathering and problem definition and negotiation will be likely to come at the beginning of treatment, and will very often be enshrined in something called an 'assessment interview', the skilful interviewer combines assessment with the other elements of interviewing in a sympathetic way.

Assessment occupies a key role within the nursing process. In an early description, Crow (1979) describes the role of assessment as the gathering of information about clients and the use of such information to identify and validate client problems. This initial stage is seen as of prime importance, since, without it, there can be no comprehensive intervention, and care will thereby be impeded. Accuracy and comprehensiveness appeared as crucial issues in assessment interviewing, in much the same way that we noticed their importance in the self-assessment implicit in reflection during the previous chapter.

However, Crow's writing focussed principally on the ill person and the effects of illness. As a result, the accuracy and comprehensiveness required related mainly to client difficulties. Other writers (e.g. Barker, 1982) have stressed the need to assess the person in a way which also allows examination of her strengths, and have also emphasized more strongly the importance of the developing relationship between nurse and client in this stage of the nursing process, much as we discussed above. These two strands (holism and relatedness) have become dominant features in recent descriptions of assessment in the nursing process, and are consistent with CB attempts to examine and deal with a range of human experiences, including health problems. Nevertheless, it is important to remember that the assessment, at least in CB approaches, is *primarily* a problem-centred (or need-centred) exercise. The client would not have come to our attention, under most circumstances, without having identified some health-related need, and the problem-oriented nature of both the nursing process and CB interviewing acknowledge that fact, and the resultant expectation of the client that such needs will be addressed as the first concern of the clinician. So, paradoxically, Crow's early formulation of assessment in the nursing process, may turn out to be the most client-centred, in the sense of responding to the client's expectations about the roles of clinician and client. Assessment remains, therefore, part of a problem-oriented nursing process, and relationship-building and investigation of the client's strengths and general personhood become aspects of enabling client and clinician to work together in addressing problems in the most effective way possible.

At this point, it is necessary to return to the idea of nursing models. In the introductory chapter, I noted that our examination of interviewing would not expressly ally itself to any particular model of nursing, and also suggested both scepticism about the empirical support *any* nursing models had received and a preference for the expressions 'nursing beliefs' or 'nursing frameworks'. Before we go on to examine the CB approach to interviewing (which, as we noted in Chapter 1, *does* embody a model of human experience which attempts to lend itself to testing), it should be acknowledged that many people are using nursing models in a variety of nursing settings. If the CB approach to interviewing is to be useful to you, then it must be sufficiently robust to allow its use within a range of nursing frameworks. Later in this chapter, I shall examine the ideas of this approach as a set of *general* propositions about human experience. By their general nature, I suggest that they are in some way superordinate to nursing models or frameworks. In the exercises, you are invited to examine how the CB approach fits in with your current practice. As a step in this direction, I shall now briefly examine the role of assessment in a well-known nursing model, and outline how it is different from and similar to CB formulations of human experience, before introducing the approach to interviewing associated with such formulations.

Roper *et al.*'s (1980) 'Activities of Living' model is widely used in the UK, and essentially views each human as an 'amalgam of activities', motivated by heirarchically defined needs. I shall refer to this model, for the rest of this chapter, as the AL model. Assessment involves data collection regarding the occurrence of each of the 12 activities in a particular individual, with emphasis on the role of the nurse in helping the client to achieve appropriate expression of activities which have been disrupted by client problems. This is seen as a continuous process, during which emphasis may shift between concentration on one or more of the activities. There is, however, little emphasis in the model on cause and effect relationships. For example, there is little discussion of how a need comes to be expressed through a given activity, how disruption occurs, or how specific nursing interventions work to address such disruptions. Equally, there is little examination of the interactions between the various activities, how these contribute to client difficulties, and how intervention by the nurse with one activity might affect other activities. These shortcomings weaken the framework in terms of its power to predict human behaviour in response to illness and to nursing intervention. In this sense, the AL approach is perhaps best described as a systematic description of a number of domains of human experience. Its associated assessments, therefore, will, by their nature, be largely descriptive and categorical. This is in itself useful, and offers a clear way of describing and recording client difficulties, but the lack of predictive power and tendency to encourage thinking in discrete categories limits its utility.

In many ways, the CB model of assessment will be familiar to the many British nurses who have been trained in the context of the AL approach, since both seek to build up a coherent picture of human experience through the use of a number of categories. Equally, both concentrate, to a large extent, on observable behaviour. There are, however, some quite major general differences, which should be understood before proceeding to examine this approach to assessment in detail. First, the CB approach is aimed at making testable predictions about client behaviour and experience, as well as describing it, and these predictions are based on a theoretical standpoint – social learning theory in its broadest sense (Bandura, 1977a). Here it has more in common with other models, for example Johnson's (1968), than with the AL model. The predictions include:

Predictions about how clients will act in given situations (e.g. when afraid, grieving, in pain).
Predictions about the effects of such acts on the client's life in general.
Predictions about the effects these actions will have on clients if no changes in trend occur (either by chance or through intervention).
Predictions about the effects of nursing interventions on client difficulties.

Whilst it is true that the AL model also attempts to draw conclusions of this kind in an implicit way, the difference between it and the CB approach is that the latter attempts to form its predictions in a more specific and testable way. This emphasis on testability and specificity is embodied in the assessment process.

Second, although the CB approach does have this theoretical underpinning, it is more appropriate to regard this as a dominant theme within the discipline, rather than an all-embracing set of rules about human nature. In fact, the CB approach is a fairly loose set of ideas about human experience and difficulty, which are shared by quite divergent trends within the discipline. I have suggested elsewhere (Newell & Dryden, 1991) that it is best to talk of a cognitive-behavioural *orientation* which comprises the following characteristics:

Basis in empirical observation.
Emphasis on individual differences.
Emphasis on human behavioural and cognitive learning.
Principle of person's ability both to shape and be shaped by the environment (mutual reciprocity).

Thus, the CB approach is eclectic rather than prescriptive in its examination of client experiences, and, unlike the AL model is not a single approach to such experiences. Third, the CB model is concerned with interactions between the categories of human experience it aims to describe. In fact, it is very often interactions of this kind that are deemed to be behind many of the difficulties with which clients present, and therefore, many of the predictions which the CB model makes are based upon them. As an example, the CB model *explicitly* hypothesizes that the client experiencing pain does so because of the influence of autonomic experiences of anxiety on muscle tone. The resulting pain experiences offer feedback to the person which contribute to negative thinking about her ability to cope. These negative thoughts themselves increase anxiety, and so the circle of increasing pain continues (Lethem *et al.*, 1983). It is easy to generate similar interactive formulations about many client experiences, for example: the effect of anxiety on clients during hospitalization (Webb, 1983), or the effect of behavioural avoidance upon body image (Newell, 1991). The issue is that, in CB formulations of human distress, the difficulties clients experience only rarely reside in one or more particular subsystems of the AL model. It is more likely that disturbances occur as a result of *interactions* between the much broader categories the CB approach describes. As a result, assessment is concerned with teasing out both disturbed performance within these broad subsystems, and in the interactions between them.

THE COGNITIVE–BEHAVIOURAL APPROACH TO ASSESSMENT

In the introductory chapter, we looked at some general background to the CB approach and to cognitive-behaviour therapy, and we have now looked at the relationship of the CB approach to one model of nursing. At this point, it is important to offer some precise characteristics of CB assessment principles. For the rest of this chapter, we shall explore one particular variant of the CB approach – the three systems model (Lang, 1971). Once again, it worth noting that this variant is only a *template* for your own interviews, not a format to be followed slavishly. Most of the remarks in this chapter relate to the gathering of information to assess the *presenting problem only*, although, there are also general guidelines regarding more general life history taking, based on CB principles of the *process* of interviewing, but not upon such principles as they relate to content.

In the previous section, I implicitly described the interactions between the three systems of the three systems model, during our discussion of the client with pain. This model examines human experience in the context of three very broad systems and their interactions. These systems, the *a*utonomic/physical system, the *b*ehavioural system and the *c*ognitive system, are said to interact to mediate client difficulties, and offer the clinician a framework in which to examine these difficulties, giving rise to the description 'ABC Model of Assessment'. The autonomic/physical system refers to bodily sensations of all kinds, but not to constructs based upon such sensations. For example, measures and client reports of rapid pulse, palpitations and nausea are evidence of imbalance within the autonomic/physical system, but client descriptions of 'anxiety' are not. Similarly, descriptions of muscular tension in the neck are physiological descriptions, whilst the self-report 'I feel tense' is not. Investigation of the behavioural system requires observation or precise description of what the client does and does not do. Again, this is to be distinguished from what the client *feels* they could or could not do under any given circumstances. Finally, the cognitive system refers to the client's self-reports of the thoughts which pass through their minds in connection with their difficulties. Once again, what is required here is reporting of what the client actually thinks, rather than what they think about their thoughts, so:

'I think all sorts of hopeless thoughts. I feel I am not worth anything'

are not sufficiently explicit, whilst:

'I think "I am a hopeless person"'

and:

'I think "everyone thinks I am worthless"'

offer sufficient information to allow us to discover exactly what the client is thinking. Later writers (e.g. Kirk, 1989) have added a fourth system to their assessments – the affective system. This refers to people's descriptions of their mood states. Whilst there is some evidence from information-processing studies (e.g. Sutherland *et al.*, 1982; Brewin, 1988) that emotions may exist as a separate system of human experience, and may be activated separately from the other systems described here, many behaviourists deny the existence of such a separate system, preferring to think of affect or emotion as a construct, in much the same way as I suggested about anxiety earlier in this section. These constructs are derived from our awareness of complex interactions between the three systems, and are best understood by a thorough investigation of each system. According to this account, the introduction of further systems confuses rather than clarifies our understanding of client experiences. Since this is particularly likely to be the case when the information offered is vague, as much of the information offered about affective states tends to be, I shall retain the more conservative analysis, and examine affect within the context of the three systems. It should be noted, however, that this is not a denial of people's *experience* of affective states, of which, as in the experience of pain, they are the best judges. It is merely a different way of searching for the detail and uniqueness of such experiences. The notion of a separate system mediating affect is rejected because, at present, this higher level description does not add to our understanding of the experience, other than giving it a label, any more than does the reductionist alternative (for example, saying that emotion *is* a series of chemical changes within the brain). There is nothing *wrong* with either the high or low level description of emotion, for it certainly is true both that people experience themselves as having sets of states which they describe as emotions, and that when they do so chemical changes are associated with such states. It is simply that the information available to the nurse from conceptualizing emotions in such ways is likely to be both limited and unhelpful.

As you have probably grasped from the above, the keynote of CB assessment using the three systems model (and this is true of other CB assessments, too) is precision. We shall return to this theme many times, but never more so than during this chapter. This emphasis on precision reflects the commitment of CB approaches to the uniqueness of each individual, a commitment they share with many nursing models and the nursing process, and which also derives from the emphasis of such approaches on testing their assumptions about human experience.

The other broad notion about humans embodied in the CB approach, their ability to be shaped by, to learn from and to shape their environment, also gives rise to the clinician's search for detail. It reflects the assertion in CB formulations of human difficulty that it is necessary to understand the precise maintaining and initiating factors in the client's environment in order to be able to help that person to effect change in her life. Assessment is, as a result, also characterized by an emphasis on such factors, and this is in turn reflected by investigation of events which precisely surround the occurrence of events the client finds problematic. Here another set of ABCs is sought, reflecting the antecedents, behaviour and beliefs, and consequences of an action (O'Leary & Wilson, 1975). These notions are quite simple. Antecedents are those occurrences which occur immediately before a problematic episode, behaviour and beliefs (the latter sometimes being investigated under the heading of 'cognitions') refer to the episode itself and the clients perceptions of it, and consequences are events immediately following a problematic episode. In each case, the interviewer uses the three systems framework to examine what occurred, with the aim of attempting to discover how the problematic behaviour is being maintained. To take the example of a client with chronic pain, the nurse might investigate a series of pain episodes in order to build up a picture of the client's responses. Here the nurse seeks links between what the client was doing beforehand, which might have precipitated the painful episode, examines precisely what the client does when pain occurs, which might have prolonged the painful experience, and investigates what happened after the event which might have reinforced inappropriate coping tactics by the client. In each case, the autonomic/physical, behavioural and cognitive systems are examined.

A detailed account of how behaviourists came to describe the mediating influences of antecedents and consequences of a behaviour upon that behaviour are beyond the scope of this book, and, indeed, it is recognized by most nurses, and by people as a whole, that events which occur close together in time often have some causal links. Equally, most nurses are aware of the general concepts of classical and operant conditioning which are though to mediate such causal links. For the present, a detailed understanding of such concepts is not needed. To understand the background to the CB approach, it is necessary to accept only three general concepts, each of which offers an incomplete account of human experience, but which, taken together, account for a great deal of such experience. These are the processes of habituation, classical conditioning and operant conditioning. Although these are complicated ideas, each can be summarized as in Figure 4.1.

In addition to accepting these three concepts, it is helpful if you can also agree, from our general experiences of life, that we are influenced by, rewarded by and learn from the experiences of others. For those wishing to find out more about conditioning processes, Stephen Walker (1984) has a very readable introduction, as well as a much more detailed examination of both the strengths and weaknesses of conditioning theories (Walker, 1987).

Habituation	The tendency of an organism to cease to respond to a repeatedly presented stimulus (e.g. the tendency of phobic clients to cease to fear after repeated exposure to the feared object).
Classical conditioning	The tendency for responses to an object or situation to become associated with other objects or situations which have been paired with it (e.g. the tendency for a child who is frightened of injections to also come to fear entering the nurse's waiting room).
Operant conditioning	The tendency for behaviours which have been rewarded (either by giving a desired stimulus or by removing an undesired one) to increase in frequency, and the tendency for responses which have been punished (either by giving an undesired stimulus or withdrawing a desired one) to decrease in frequency.

Figure 4.1 Conditioning processes

AIMS OF ASSESSMENT

In the above clinical example, the nurse aims to find out, through the use of the two ABCs, the defining characteristics of the individual's pain experiences. At this point let me introduce the concepts of *necessity* and *sufficiency*. The nurse, in examining the client's problems, is looking only for those characteristics of the client which are necessary and sufficient to account for the client's difficulties. This search may be quite far-reaching, but is based both on the need to cover all those aspects of the client's life which bear upon the problem and help to either maintain it or cope with it (sufficiency), and to exclude those aspects of the client's life which do not (necessity). Although the concept of necessity may seem strange, apparently reducing the client to *just* the problem, the aim here is threefold: to avoid muddying the waters of assessment by examining elements which are not relevant to the client's problem, to avoid wasted time for both client and nurse and to preserve the client's dignity and privacy by intruding as little as possible into extraneous parts of her life. No doubt a good deal of more general information does come to light during the course of assessment, but this does not need to be focussed on by the nurse (although it always needs to be acknowledged with the client), who attempts to keep structure in the interview. By so doing, she seeks to achieve the first aim of the assessment interview: *to gain the information necessary and sufficient to arrive at an understanding of the client's difficulties.* Clearly in some circumstances, this will not be completely possible during a first meeting, or even by interview alone. Nevertheless, the nurse should have sufficient idea of the nature of the client's difficulties to (a) be able to say whether her interventions are likely to benefit the client, (b) decide what further assessment strategies (e.g. diary-keeping by the client, a period of observation, a further information-gathering session) are required, and (c) transmit these findings to the client, whether this be by offering a rationale for treatment or negotiating further information-gathering strategies.

A second aim for assessment is the *commencement of the therapeutic liaison*. Of course, this is of great importance if the nurse and client are to work together to resolve the client's difficulties over any extended period of time, and the assessment interview, which is a often a first meeting, sets the scene as to how that relationship will continue. A great deal of the material in Chapter 2 demonstrates how the nurse can begin to establish this relationship at the outset of an initial interview. As information-gathering begins, however, this process can continue and deepen, with the use of appropriate skills by the nurse. However, even if the assessment interview is likely to be the only time the nurse and client meet, the establishment of rapport is still of crucial importance, since such trust will enhance the transfer of information between the client and nurse. Paradoxically, the building of a therapeutic alliance during a single meeting may be even more crucial than during the first of a series of meetings. The nurse has only one attempt to transmit information to the client at such one-off meetings, and also only a single opportunity to give the client impressions about the nature of the nurse–client relationship. Both these issues are important for the client's progress during the course of her health care. If the nurse has been asked to offer only a single consultation, or if she has assessed the client and felt her own interventions would be unsuitable, and intends to refer the client elsewhere, the handling of such meetings needs some sensitivity. Ideally, the client goes away from the interview with information, hope, and positive expectations about the conduct of health care consultations in the future. In this way, the nurse attempts to enhance the likelihood that other interviewers in the future will get as useful information as possible from the client, and that the client, in her turn, will be as likely as possible to be at ease in future consultations, because of her past positive experiences of the *process* of the interview, even if the outcome was not necessarily what she would have wished. We cannot help all clients, but we can transmit this fact to them sensitively, and in such a way as to maximize the likelihood that someone else can.

A specific subcomponent of general relationship-building is the *orientation* of the client to the nurse's therapeutic approach. This is important both for the generation of compliance and so as to enable the client to offer informed consent to treatment. Many nursing interventions require the client to carry out a range of nursing instructions away from the interview setting, whether these instructions have been offered in a didactic fashion or, as is generally preferred in modern health care, through serial negotiations with the client. In Chapter 6 we shall be discussing compliance in rather more detail, and indeed, the generation of such compliance is a key element of all stages of the nurse–client relationship. At assessment, however, it is certainly important that the client has a clear idea of how the nurse is accustomed to work, and the theoretical underpinnings of any advice she might be likely to offer in the future.

It is often suggested in clinical practice that clients are uninterested in complicated explanations of how treatment works, and would prefer to leave this to the clinician. Whilst this may be true of some clients, this may well reflect their past experiences of health care, and the punishing consequences of asking for information from remote health care professionals. In any event, the finding that, in general, clients want to know as much as possible about their diagnosis and the associated treatments is an extremely durable one in the medical psychology literature, dating back to extremely early studies (summarized in Ley, 1977). It is also worth commenting that to *assume* that clients are uninterested in their own care, may well have less to do with the needs of the client than those of the clinician, who may feel threatened both by the idea of the knowledgeable client and the practical skills needed for accurate information-giving. This view also violates a number of assumptions about the client discussed in Chapter 1, for example, clients being skilled, desiring change, desiring interaction, being like us.

Even if it were the case that clients would rather leave the details of treatment to us, as clinicians, to sort out, the issue of informed consent is still a compelling reason for offering a detailed orientation to the therapeutic interventions on offer. Clearly it is impossible to consent to something about which one knows nothing, or understands in only the most hazy fashion. Once again, the counter-argument has been made that clients can never have the kind of understanding of treatment that the clinician possesses. This is very confused thinking, confounding (a) theoretical and practical understanding and (b) form and content. In the first case, it is possible to have a very high degree of theoretical knowledge of a subject, and very little practical knowledge, or the reverse, as in the examples of the expert garage mechanic who can strip down an engine and repair it with ease, but has only the sketchiest of ideas about the electrical principles of the working of a spark plug, and the physicist who understands such principles with more precision than any other scientist, but doesn't know one end of a plug spanner from the other. One form of knowledge is not higher or better than the other, both have appropriateness in their own arenas. Similar examples are the improvising jazz musician who cannot read musical notation and the classical musician who, if called upon to improvise so much as a single line, is like a beginner again. The issue here is one of the *kind* of information the client needs, not the level, and here, the principles of precision, completeness and practicality are useful guides. As to who decides on what the constituents of these three principles are, the job of the nurse is to gather the client's views on these matters, in the same way that she would collect any other piece of assessment information.

The second issue, that of form and content, is also one of information transmission, and simply states that the most complicated information may be expressed in simple words without any loss of content or clarity. With regard both to this emphasis on the possibility of clear communication of complex information and the necessity of offering information specific to each client's requirements, I suggest that both are issues of respect and time for the client. They are also both of immense practical importance to the nurse, because of their relationship to compliance. My own experience, and that of most therapists in the CB tradition, is that clients generally both desire and need a great deal of information about the rationale and the conduct of treatment, and readily grasp such details when sufficient care is taken in their transmission. They also appreciate the hidden message such communications offer about respect for and alliance with the client.

We have already noted that this chapter is primarily concerned with assessment of the client's main presenting difficulties. Nevertheless, assessment also contains elements of *general history-taking*, which attempt to set the client in her more general context, and to elicit any elements of her history which have particular bearing on the presenting difficulties. Although such general history taking should be complete, the CB view is that it should not receive great emphasis, since this would detract from concentration on the client's difficulties in the present, those aspects of present circumstances which serve to maintain them, and planning for their future moderation. Even outside cognitive-behaviourism, many orientations within nursing stress the importance of the here-and-now in the examination of client difficulties. CB assessment seeks to demonstrate this emphasis to the client through direct experience of how the interview is conducted. Thus, the message conveyed to the client through the process of the interview (as well as by direct statements, in many cases) is: 'It's what's happening to you now that is important'. This has a good deal of congruence with Dillon's (1990) description of client agendas in clinical interviews, where their preoccupations are generally concerns about their social, personal and economic worlds, and the consequences for these worlds of their presenting difficulties.

Towards the end of the assessment phase, the client is introduced to the concepts of *goal-setting and planning*. Goal-setting and planning fulfil several purposes at assessment. The client is offered further opportunities to participate in and negotiate her care, and the balance between nurse activity, which has been quite high in the early stages of the assessment interview because of her need to elicit information from the client, and client activity alters, with client participation increasing. This aims to create for the client the expectation of further increased participation as treatment continues. The process of goal-setting is also a first major experience for the client of negotiation between herself and the nurse, as both seek to define together the nature of the clients difficulties, the associated goals and in what ways both client and nurse will act in order to move the client between the problem-state and the goal-state. In this way, the nurse offers the client a 'taster' of what the process of treatment will be like.

Closely related to goal-setting is the concept of *measurement*. This is crucial to the CB orientation, and has become increasingly accepted as a key element in many areas of nursing. Again, at assessment, the nurse offers the client a foretaste of how measurement will affect her through the course of the therapeutic relationship, by explaining its relevance and conduct, and doing practical measurement exercises together during the course of defining and refining the problem. Numerous writers have published rating scales of problem severity (e.g. Marks, 1986), and these can serve as templates for use with clients in a wide variety of settings. In addition, some of the rating scales used to examine specific areas of functioning (e.g. Melzack, 1975) can form part of a measurement package. At this point in treatment, the nurse can also use the concept of measurement to reinforce the notion of client improvement, and stress the value to both client and nurse of feedback on client performance as a means of assessing treatment progress, tailoring the interventions to the client's individual needs, offering the client rewarding evidence and negotiating adjustments to the interventions where necessary. Such measurements may also at this time form part of *baseline information* recording strategies, the role and importance of which are again discussed with the client.

The aims we have discussed above can be summarized as in Figure 4.2. Each aim can be associated with a number of nurse and client objectives. In this case, I am suggesting a number of behavioural outcomes for the nurse and the client, which represent things which the nurse and the client will be able to do by the end of the interview, as a result of what has occurred during the course of the interview. These sorts of objective are common in educational circles (at least those which are concerned with *outcome* more than with the process of education (Quinn, 1988)), and represent goals for both client and nurse which we could test out and measure at the end of the assessment session, should we so wish. The degree of precision and formality with which such outcomes are examined varies from individual to individual and from occasion to occasion. Nevertheless, most commentators on the interviewing process are agreed both on the need for objectives and the need for some kind of evaluation of our success in achieving them. A number of sample objectives is offered in Figure 4.3. In the context of supervision of beginning clinicians, the nurse's objectives might well have the additional use of forming a template for evaluating the learner's interviewing expertise.

Having looked at what we hope to achieve during assessment interviewing, we will now go on to examine *how* to achieve those aims. Thus, the next section describes what kind of information we shall seek during the assessment interview, and is followed in Chapter 5 by an examination of how to go about getting this information.

To gain the information *necessary and sufficient* to arrive at an understanding of the client's difficulties and formulate a plan of care.

Commencement of the therapeutic liaison.

Orientation of the client to the types of intervention to be offered.

General history-taking

Goal setting and planning

Measurement

Baseline information

Figure 4.2 Aims of assessment

By the end of the interview, the *nurse* will be able to:

State the client's main problem(s).

State and justify a formulation of the client's difficulties, with due regard to causative and maintaining factors.

Describe a plan of care or other arrangements negotiated with the client.

Describe the client's responses to the nurse's description of the rationale and plan of care, including issues of consent.

State and justify her view of the current state of the therapeutic relationship.

Relate the client's difficulties to relevant issues from the client's general history.

Show what baseline measures have been taken and/or describe what tactics for measurement have been negotiated with the client for the future.

By the end of the interview, the *client* will be able to:

Describe the nurse's formulation of her difficulties.

State the rationale for these difficulties and for intervention offered by the nurse.

Describe the plan of care or other arrangements negotiated with the nurse.

Describe the role of evaluation and measurement in the plan of care.

Describe what measures were used with the nurse, or what tactics for future measurement were negotiated.

Figure 4.3 Objectives at assessment

THE COMPONENTS OF ASSESSMENT – NECESSARY AND SUFFICIENT INFORMATION ABOUT THE MAIN PROBLEM

This section seeks to answer the question: 'What things do I ask about in order to determine the nature of the client's difficulties?' This will be examined within the context of the CB description of assessment offered earlier, describing the course of examining each set of ABCs, and the questioning required to elicit detailed information in each case. The nurse usually allows the client to set the agenda by means of an open question, which elicits from the client some general statement of the problem, giving the nurse the opportunity of continuing the interview by inquiry about more specific areas of difficulty, associated with each of the three systems. Examples of clients with difficulty in rising from a chair, owing to painful arthritic joints, inability to sleep and difficulty climbing stairs owing to breathlessness, will be used for illustrative purposes.

Autonomic/physical system

Here, the nurse examines physical difficulties which are contributing to the client's current health problems. Often, nurses are preoccupied with such physical symptoms, and have adopted a medically oriented 'systems of life' approach (e.g. respiratory system, gastrointestinal system, etc.) as a way of guiding their questioning. Clients, of course, do not divide their bodies in precisely this way, and may find such an approach disjointed. As an alternative, cognitive-behaviourists prefer general questions which reflect client conceptualizations of their difficulties.

It is expected that such questions will lead the interviewer towards a coverage of relevant elements of the various bodily systems, as does serial questioning about the role of each such system, but preserve the client's perceived control of the interview, since she can answer in her own way. It is the nurse's job to retain cognitively the structure she requires in order to assimilate the information, not to overload the client with a questioning regime which springs from this structure but whose significance is opaque to the client. Thus, a key early question is:

'Can you tell me what happens to you physically?'

This question is asked with regard to the antecedents of problematic episodes, the episodes themselves and their consequences:

Antecedents:

'Can you tell me what happens to you physically just *before* you start to move out of the chair?'

Behaviour:

'Can you tell me what happens to you physically when you *are* in bed and trying to get to sleep?'

Consequences:

'Can you tell me what happens to you physically *after* you have stopped trying to walk upstairs?'

Responses from the client are then followed by the nurse in a structured way, as she attempts to quantify each response. Here, the most relevant question forms are those which specify the response, state the frequency of the response, state the severity of the response, state the duration of the response, and state the modifiers of the response. These questions are asked in the context of antecedents, the episode itself, and consequences:

Antecedents:

'How would you describe this feeling?'

'When you try to get up, how many time during the attempt would you get the feeling?'

'How severe . . . '

'How long would the feeling last?'

'Does anything make it better or worse?'

Behaviour:

'How many times during the night do you feel these physical sensations when you are trying to get to sleep?'

or:

'How many times on an average night would you get these feelings?'

and:

'How long . . . '

and so on.

Consequences:

'How often do you find that the pain goes away after you have stopped trying to walk upstairs?'

'How long does it take for the pain to go away?'

'How severe is the pain when you start walking again?'

Clearly, the above shows a very close, precise style of questioning, and clients may be unused to being invited to give answers which involve them in considering their responses in such detail. As a result, they may require a good deal of prompting, and the nurse may guide them towards the most accurate answers that can be expected *under the present circumstances:*

'On average?'

'Roughly?'

'Round about?'

'Most of the time?'

'Always?'

'More than ten?'

Even though what has been presented above is a highly stylized account, which is humanized in the clinical examples offered at the end of Chapter 5 and in Appendix 2, there remains, in such a focal style of interviewing, naturally, an issue here of hectoring the client, and this is a mistake commonly made by beginning interviewers of all disciplines. In Chapter 5, when we examine the process of assessment interviewing, and also in Chapter 7, when we discuss emotion handling, we shall investigate how to minimize the danger of badgering the client. Having examined the basic questioning associated with the autonomic/ physical system, let us now turn to the behavioural and cognitive systems. Indeed, it must be said that the questions are almost the same, since the other two systems are approached in a way identical to the first, as the need for precision is equally important in all three systems.

Behavioural system

The nurse now attempts to elicit what precisely the client does when the problematic episodes occur. Valuable information can be gained about the client's coping tactics (both adaptive and maladaptive) during this section of the interview, and the nurse is also able to build a firmer picture of the effect of the client's difficulties upon her life as a whole. However, at this stage, the questioning remains focal to the presenting problem.

The key orienting question here is:

'What do you actually do?'

Thus, in the context of antecedents, behaviour (the actual occurrence of the problematic episode) and consequences, this is translated into:

Antecedents:

'What do you actually do before you try to get out of the chair?'

Behaviour (occurrence of the problematic episode):

'What do you actually do when you are in bed trying to get to sleep?'

Consequences:

'What do you actually do after you have tried to walk up the stairs?'

The probe questions which follow these general openings are much the same as for the autonomic/physical system, and so we will just examine a couple of further examples:

'How many cups of tea would you make during an average night?'

'How long would you sit at the top of the stairs for?'

'How severe would the back pain be after rising from the chair?'

Cognitive system

Finally, the nurse examines the thinking and beliefs of the client regarding each problematic episode. Generally, this includes some examination of the client's mood states at such times. Examination of client cognitions helps the nurse understand their contribution to the maintenance of the problem, since this kind of 'self-talk' is associated with changes in mood, bodily functioning and behaviour (e.g. Beck, 1976). In CB terms, the nurse is looking for evidence that the client's thoughts are acting as either rewards or punishments for the client.

Here, the question form is:

'What do you think?'

and the nurse might begin with the following to investigate antecedents, behavioural episode and consequences:

'What do you think about before you have to rise from the chair?'

'What do you think about when you are trying to get to sleep?'

What do you think about after you have tried to climb the stairs?'

A supplementary question may help the client to tap the affective components of these thoughts (e.g. 'How does that make you feel?').

At this point, you should be able to describe the probe questions associated with the cognitive system antecedent, behavioural episode and consequence questions stated above, in terms of frequency, severity, and so on. Also consider asking questions about the client's beliefs about what is happening during an episode and the associated fears about what *might* happen.

Further examination of the ABCs – specifying the problem

After the above questions, the nurse should have a detailed picture of typical problem episodes. This does not, however, yet capture the role of these episodes within the client's life. According to Bandura's (1977b) principle of mutual reciprocity, it is to be expected that the client's difficulties will affect other areas of her life, and that she herself will affect the course of her difficulties. The above sections have sought out cause and effect relationships which occur at the time of each episode *within the client*. In order to understand fully, however, the factors maintaining the problem, an exploration of external factors is also required, relating to typical problem episodes, but also to the client's experiences more generally. The result, hopefully, is a picture both of how external circumstances affect the client's difficulties, and how those difficulties themselves affect the client's interactions with the world at large. Questions which specify the problem in this way also have the advantage of keeping to the CB agenda of focussing primarily on the *client's concerns*, which, as we have noted in earlier chapters, are often more to do with social, external functioning than with medical notions of physical health.

We will now examine a series of questions which specify the circumstances under which problematic episodes occur, offer clues as to why such episodes occur, and define the impact of the episodes on the client's life.

Richards & MacDonald (1990) have offered one structure of questioning – *the five Ws* – which goes a long way towards defining the problem in the kind of detail we require, and have set this structure into the context of a behavioural analysis based on the three systems model. This kind of approach has been adopted by numerous other CB writers, and consists of investigation of *what* the problem is, *where* and *when* it occurs, *with whom* it occurs and *why* it occurs. To this list, we would do well to add one further W – *what do others do* when the problem occurs.

Our analysis of the three systems has already given a clear picture of many aspects of the first of these *six* Ws, describing with precision what the problematic event is on each occurrence, with reference to each of the three systems, so we can now examine *where* the problem occurs by use of the following questions:

'Where are you when the difficulty occurs?'

Here the attempt by the nurse is to establish exactly what environmental variables make the problem better or worse, and so the opening question is followed by a series of relevant probe questions. In the case of our first client example these might be:

'Are some chairs better than others?'

'Is the problem better in some situations than others?'

Thus, the interviewer might learn that the problem only ever occurs in restaurants or at meal times at home, and that the chairs involved have no arms, providing valuable information about what is maintaining the problem.

The next question – *when* does the problem occur – expects answers from the client about regular variation according to time of day, day of the week, and season of the year, but is also a further question about antecedents and consequences. We have already asked the client what happens before problematic events, because we assume there will be some causal link between the antecedents of events and the events themselves. However, by asking the question again, in a different manner and context, we offer the client an additional chance to make such causal links. So, as well as replies about time of day, etc., we should also expect responses which indicate other behaviours which habitually precede or follow the problematic events. Finally, we should be alert for replies which have a temporal basis which is irregular but predictable, as in the case of women suffering with premenstrual syndrome, who can reliably tie their difficulties to a particular phase in the menstrual cycle, even when the cycle itself is not regular, or the grieving person who ties feeling particularly low to 'anniversaries' which are not regular throughout the calendar.

In investigating *with whom* the problematic episode occurs, we are principally concerned with what effect the presence of such persons has upon the client's difficulties, and it is for this reason that I have added the notion of *what such people do*, since most of the probe questions which follow the initial:

'Can you tell me who is present when . . . ?'

question will relate to the interactions between the client and these others. Here we can investigate the behaviour of such others in exactly the way we would examine that of the client – in terms of the three systems. We do not have direct access to their thoughts and physical feelings, but we can examine them in an analogical way, by asking the client, for example, what the people around her *said*, this being representative in some degree of thought, and how they seemed *physically* (perhaps angrily or anxiously aroused), as well as their *behaviour*. So we have some idea, from the client, of how those around her respond during the problematic incidents. We can also ask about how their responses to the client related to antecedents and consequences, as well as to the behaviour itself. Finally, we can investigate the client's own responses to the behaviour of others in the problem situations, again using ABCs.

Finally, in our series of Ws, we come to the most difficult question of all. *Why* does the problematic episode occur? Once again, cognitive-behaviourism acknowledges the power and knowledge of the client in defining and understanding her own problems, and so her assessment of maintaining factors is extremely important. Here, the client has an opportunity to express those views directly, along with any fears she may have about what is happening to her. An understanding of the client's views is also important when designing intervention strategies. Many writers have discussed the difficulty involved in asking the question 'why', and, indeed, it must be admitted that such a question is both threatening to the client and often difficult to answer. It can, however, be avoided, or 'softened', whilst retaining the same sense:

'Perhaps you have views about what is maintaining the problem?'

'Are there ideas you have yourself about the cause of the difficulty?'

and so on. Sometimes, however, it may be important to ask the 'why' question directly, however, and we shall discuss how to go about this in the section on the process of assessment interviewing.

Having reviewed the six Ws, we can now turn to a few final questions which round off our appreciation of the impact of the problem on the client's life. The first two, those of frequency and duration, we have discussed already, with relation to ABCs, but they are asked again in this more general context since we want to know not only how frequent particular symptoms are on each problematic occasion (as sought during our analysis of ABCs), but also how frequently episodes occur, and how long ago the problem started. With regard to *duration*, we also have the opportunity to examine the circumstances at *onset* of the problem, any *fluctuations*, and any previous attempts at *coping* with the problem which the client has made, including *formal treatments* of one kind or another. Again, the ABC model can be used as a way of approaching the specific variables associated with variability of the problem in the past. Both these questions offer some idea of the impact on the client's life, particularly when combined with the information we already have about the severity of the problem. Finally, we may ask a general question about impact on the client's life:

'Can you describe how the problem affects your day to day living?'

As well as helping us gauge the seriousness of the problem in terms of handicap to the client's life, this also provides information about the client's likely *goals* from intervention. We may also ask about these explicitly, as a prelude to the formal process of goal-setting.

This concludes our examination of how cognitive-behaviourists arrive at a picture of the elements of the client's problems which are necessary and sufficient to gain an understanding of those difficulties and organize and negotiate interventions with that client. The main components of assessment are shown in Figure 4.4, and are best remembered by the mnemonic ABCS:

(A)NTECEDENTS

    (A)utonomic/physical
    (B)ehavioural
    (C)ognitive

(B)EHAVIOURAL EVENT

    (A)utonomic/physical
    (B)ehavioural
    (C)ognitive

(C)ONSEQUENCES

    (A)utonomic/physical
    (B)ehavioural
    (C)ognitive

(S)PECIFIERS

    What?
    Where?
    When?
    Who with?
    What do others do?
    Why?
    (five/six Ws)
    How often do episodes occur?
    How long ago did episodes begin?
    How do episodes affect the client's daily life?
    What goals does the client have from treatment?

Figure 4.4 Components of cognitive-behavioural interviewing

(A)utonomic/physical
(B)ehavioural
(C)ognitive for:
(A)ntecedents
(B)ehavioural episode
(C)onsequences
(S)pecifiers

Of course, it may be argued that this format is not sufficiently exhaustive. For instance, we have not mentioned any questions regarding drugs and alcohol, interpersonal relationships, personality variables which might affect the problem, health beliefs, an so on. This is only partly true. We have not mentioned *specific questions* which elicit this information, and, indeed if we had done this for every

(A)NTECEDENTS

(A)utonomic/physical – location of pain before a task is performed, description of pain, level of pain, measurement of pain, autonomic anxiety symptoms, frequency and duration of symptoms.

(B)ehavioural – attempts to protect painful area (by changes of posture, etc.), other precautions, use of medication, coping tactics, what is said to others, attempts to enlist help.

(C)ognitive – thoughts of further injury, thoughts of pain, belief in inability to perform tasks, thoughts about continuing invalid status, attempts to avoid task performance, thoughts about competency as a person.

(B)EHAVIOURAL EVENT

(A)utonomic/physical – location of pain during task performance, description of pain, level of pain, measurement of pain, autonomic anxiety symptoms, frequency and duration of symptoms.

(B)ehavioural – use of six Ws to specify situations when pain occurs. Frequency, duration of painful episodes.

(C)ognitive – see antecendents.

(C)ONSEQUENCES

(A)utonomic/physical – location of pain after task performance. Particular note of diminution of pain.

(B)ehavioural – tactics to help pain diminish, changes of posture, use of analgesia, other activities after task performance/painful episode.

(C)ognitive – See antecedents.

(S)PECIFIERS

What – is person doing when pain occurs, what does person do when pain occurs, what can person do without pain, what makes it better or worse?

Where – is person when pain occurs?

When – does pain occur, time of day/month/year. Frequency, duration?

Who with?

What do others do – reassurance? offer of massage, medication, task completion on behalf of client? distraction? how are others affected by problem?

Why – does client think pain occurs? what does client think caused it?

(six Ws)

How often do episodes occur?

How long ago did episodes begin?

How do episodes affect the client's daily life – what can client not do because of problem?

Figure 4.5 Cognitive-behavioural interviewing in the pain clinic

area, this chapter would read simply as a list of questions, rather like a recipe book. However, in the main, what has been offered is a schema for the collection of information, and a good number of specific questions, which might be of

(A)NTECEDENTS

(A)utonomic/physical – physical sensations prior to a skin eruption, early changes in skin noted, anxiety symptoms noted.

(B)ehavioural – avoided/overused products/situations. Situations/substances associated with onset of an episode.

(C)ognitive – beliefs about what might cause an eruption. Fears about bodily appearance/reactions of others.

(B)EHAVIOURAL EVENT

(A)utonomic/physical – description of nature of skin during an episode. Autonomic symptoms (e.g. when in public, when bathing, putting on make-up, looking in mirror).

(B)ehavioural – avoidances when skin is disturbed (public, social situations, use of particular products). Details of performance of treatment routines. Seeking of reassurance. Precautionary measures, use of disguise tactics. Excessive behaviours (checking of skin, overuse of creams/makeup, scratching). Use six Ws.

(C)ognitive – fears about continuing/increasing disfigurement. Thoughts about reactions of others.

(C)ONSEQUENCES

(A)utonomic/physical – description of skin after an episode. Diminution of autonomic symptoms.

(B)ehavioural – resumption of avoided activities, or continuing avoidance. Continuing use of medication (any variation?) Continuing checking behaviours.

(C)ognitive – fears of further attacks. Continuing disruption of body image.

(S)PECIFIERS

What – is the nature of the disruption to the skin?
Where – is the client (always on holiday? swimming bath?)?
When – time of day/month/year (e.g. scratches in bed, when bored; always just before menstruation; always in summer)?
Who with – (e.g. never scratches when others are present)?
What do others do – evidence of stigma? sympathy? advice-giving? reassurance?
Why – client's own view of why episodes occur when they do and causative factors.
(five/six Ws)
How often do episodes occur?
How long ago did episodes begin?
How do episodes affect the client's daily life?

Figure 4.6 Cognitive-behavioural interviewing of clients with skin complaints

interest to a nurse working in one setting rather than another, can be inserted into one or other of the categories. An exhaustive and coherent examination of a client's experiences using the ABCs model should quite naturally address issues such as these, in the course of the investigation of the ABCs. Thus, medication or alcohol logically form part of our investigation of the autonomic/physical system, and may also be described by clients in terms of an antecedent, part of the behaviour, or a consequence; interpersonal relationships appear in answers to the 'who with' question; health beliefs arise in response to questioning about cognitions, and so on. To clarify this, examples of what specific areas might be addressed by nurses working in a pain clinic and in a ward specializing in skin complaints are offered in Figures 4.5 and 4.6.

This closes our discussion of the components of cognitive-behavioural interviewing. The following chapter examines how the interviewer goes about fulfilling her other objectives during assessment interviewing, most of which are concerned with skills in the process of negotiation with the client. Because of the importance of attempting to unite structure, content and process, the clinical example of assessment interviewing is given at the end of Chapter 5.

EXERCISES

1 Figures 4.5 and 4.6 offered some pointers on tailoring a CB assessment to a specific clinical setting. Examine your own clinical role, and use the format shown in Figure 4.4 to draw up a schedule of issues to be covered in the kind of client you are likely to encounter.

2 Examine several recent assessment interviews you have done, using the schedule you have drawn up to assess:

How well you have assessed the clients' difficulties in these interviews?
How far the schedule is likely to improve your ability to specify the clients' difficulties?

3 Using the schedule you have devised, enlist the help of a colleague to practise for your *next* assessment interview, then reflect upon the process using the guidelines in Chapter 3.

4 Perform the information-gathering stage of your next interview using the assessment schedule, in the light of your reflections on the practice interview in Exercise 3. Again, reflect upon your performance.

FURTHER READING

Dryden, W. & Golden, W.L. (eds) (1986) *Cognitive-behavioural Approaches to Psychotherapy*. London. Harper & Row.
Richards, D.A. & McDonald, R. (1990) *Behavioural Psychotherapy: A Handbook for Nurses*. Oxford. Heinemann.

5   The therapeutic alliance – process skills of assessment

The previous chapter concentrated very much on the *what* of interviewing, but said very little about *how* to get that information in the most sensitive way. It is with the practice of this sensitivity in relating to the client that this chapter is chiefly concerned. The second aim of the assessment interview was the beginning of the therapeutic alliance, which draws us into an examination of more than the content of the assessment interview. Here we are concerned with the best *process* by which such information may be gained, both from the point of view of ensuring optimum transfer of information, where the client has the best possible opportunity to tell her story and the nurse the best chance of being able to make sense of it, and also in order to create the best impression possible on the client, with the aim of enhancing the likelihood of a fruitful therapeutic relationship in the future. Elements related to goal-setting and negotiation, and to dealing with unusual interviews, are also dealt with in this chapter, because of the emphasis on collaboration which renders these primarily issues of process. In Chapter 2, we spent some time looking at the general skills required to open an interview effectively, focussing on introductions, links with previous experiences, setting the scene and agenda and entering into early negotiation with the client. All these are elements of relationship building which will be useful throughout treatment, because they have offered the client the opportunity to become a participant in care, either explicitly, through the offer of direct partnership, or implicitly, through acknowledging the client's rights in the care process by accepting her as an equal and by the offering of information. The assessment part of the interview builds on these beginnings by continuing to demonstrate to the client her value in treatment. Appropriate verbal and non-verbal behaviours which help the flow of information and the therapeutic alliance are those which:

Keep the client oriented and share the interviewing process with her.
Reward the client's information.
Reward the client's previous attempts at coping.

ORIENTATION OF THE CLIENT AND SHARING THE INTERVIEW

Of these three components of sensitive interviewing, the first is the most crucial, comprising of a large number of subcomponents. Orientation of the client to what is happening during the interview is a key method of showing the client her value, our dependence upon her, and our trust in her. Keeping the client clear about the conduct of every stage in the interview begins with the agenda-setting exercise we discussed in Chapter 2, and continues throughout, both through repeated description by the nurse of what is likely to occur next, and the adopting by the nurse of a coherent interview structure. As well as demonstrating respect for the client, the nurse also shows control over the interviewing process, making the client aware of her relevant expertise. The following are some key behaviours which the nurse can adopt in order to keep the client orientated during information-gathering sessions and beyond:

Proceeding from the general to the specific by means of moving from general open questions, through more specific open questions to closed questions which specify the required detail for each area of the client's difficulties. As we saw in the previous chapter, the interview as a whole generally begins with an extremely general open question (open in the sense that it leaves the door open to a whole range of client responses), such as:

'Can you tell me about the difficulties which have brought you here today.'

However, the questions which began each section of our investigation of the ABCs are also general open questions. These become more specific if we ask the client to tell us more about a particular area, and such *specific open questions* are a good tactic in getting the client to 'open up' an area:

'Could you describe in more detail what happens when you try and get up from the meal table?'

This is an open question because it still gives the client considerable leeway in answering, but specific because it specifies the general parameters (at the meal table) about which the information is sought.

When we get to the finer detail, however, closed questions are often required. Here, all but a very narrow exit for client responses are closed, and replies are therefore controlled to a great degree by the questioner. For this reason, such questions need to be used sensitively and only when necessary. Usually, closed questions admit of only yes/no answers or numbers:

'How many a times a day?'

'Do you ever . . . ?'

Clearly a long string of such questions can be intimidating, since the client has to think according to the terms stated by the interviewer. Nevertheless, closed questions are an efficient way to get the kind of quantitative information which is often required at assessment. Their intimidating character can be softened by an introduction by the nurse, again indicating the value of enlisting the client as a partner in the therapeutic process:

'Now in a second, I'm going to require a lot of intricate detail from you, so that we can both get a clear picture of how this problem affects your life. Because of this, I'm going to ask quite a string of questions, one after another. Please don't worry if these seem difficult to answer. It is what *you* think about the problem that I'm trying to get at, so stop me or slow me down, if you need to.'

This is the basic questioning sequence used in cognitive-behavioural interviewing, and seeks to capitalize on our ability to remember specifics when they are set in the context of more general information. Thus, the general open questions asked for each component of assessment (ABCs) attempts to act as a cue for the more detailed questioning to follow. This tactic of presenting general information (in this case questions) before more specific is a common tactic in education, and has been increasingly recognized in medical interviewing.

It is not necessary, however, to always use the interrogative form in order to gain information from the client. Most *questions can be rephrased as statements*. In the context of eliciting emotion (Hobson, 1984) this is a particularly useful technique, but it can also be adapted for information gathering, especially where the nurse wishes the client to expand upon a particular topic:

'It sounds as if Sunday nights, before work on a Monday, are the most difficult times.'

Such statements can be fitted into the 'general to specific' format, retaining the benefit of orienting the client to what is likely to follow in terms of questioning form.

By contrast, although the following of a set format can help in orienting the client to the process of the interview, departure from that format is also sometimes helpful. Here the nurse attempts to *be flexible and follow client cues*. The issue of orientation here is one of *meaning*, rather than structure. Continually moving the client from one topic to another is known to be disorientating (Dillon, 1990). If the nurse can perceive and follow client cues, exploring particular areas of concern in response to the client's apparent wish to do so, yet still retain (internally) some structure to the interview, other issues can be returned to when the client is ready. As well as increasing client perception of continuity, this tactic also conveys to the client the message that it is *their* agenda that is important to the nurse. In reality, continual following of client cues during *assessment* is a difficult method for interviewers to follow entirely, and there may also be issues of difficulty for some client, who will welcome a structure within which to work. Perhaps the issue of flexibility is most important here, and a combination of both structured and cue-driven interviewing is recommended. Many interviewers go through a stage of following 'plans' of interviewing process slavishly until their confidence grows sufficiently to allow them to extemporize upon them. Such improvisation is best practised from the beginning, however, since it requires the flexibility and respect for the client which is to be sought at all times.

Having said this, it is as well to note that there are times when the interviewer needs to *redirect the client*, perhaps quite forcibly. Once again, this is about orientation. The client comes to an increasing awareness of the kind of information that is sought during assessment through the use of cues by the interviewer.

In this way, the client also gains direct experience of what the therapeutic relationship is likely to consist of, since the nurse demonstrates the focal style of working and thus offers the client the implicit choice of whether she wishes or is able to work in this way. The nurse recognizes that clients may need direction as well as space to talk and pursue themes, since time and concentration (for both nurse and client) are limited. Thus, the nurse might redirect a client with a response such as:

> 'Now, I recognize that this area is very important to you, and I hope we can return to it later. For the moment, just to keep things clear in my mind, I wonder if we can return to the topic of . . . '

This kind of redirection is also an experience of negotiation, an idea which the nurse will return to throughout treatment. Of course, it only has value it the nurse sticks to her part of the bargain and *does* return to the topic if she says she will. If the reason for redirection is a different one (for example if the client is offering a great deal of detail which threatens to swamp the nurse's concentration), the redirection itself should honestly reflect this. Once again, provided it is handled sensitively, it is an opportunity for sharing between client and nurse:

> 'I must just stop you at this stage, for a second. You are giving me very valuable information, but actually the problem is that there's just too much for me to take in all at once. Can we focus just on . . . '

In every case, the nurse attempts to share with the client any difficulties which arise during the interview. Allied to this notion of sharing power in the conduct of the interview, the nurse also *seeks feedback about both the content and process of the interview at regular intervals*, in order to assure herself both that the information she has gained has been adequately understood, and that it accurately reflects the client's desired agenda with regard both to the material covered and the amount of time allowed for that material. Here are some sample statements which indicate how the nurse can combine the goals of ensuring adequate information has been gained and engaging the client by acknowledging her knowledge of her own difficulties and desire for negotiation and interaction.

> 'Can I just check that I have understood you clearly about . . . '

> 'Let me just be sure I understand that . . . '

> 'Is there something more you need to tell me about . . . '

> 'I have the feeling there's something more . . . '

> 'Is it OK for us to pass on to talk about . . . '

Where feedback is sought particularly about content, the nurse can then go on to offer summaries and paraphrases of what the client has said, again checking regularly that these are, in fact, correct. Here the client gains additional feedback herself regarding the value to the nurse of her responses.

We have already noted that cognitive-behaviourists ask a great many questions during the course of assessment, although these may often be rephrased as statements. Therefore, the interviewer needs to pay a good deal of attention to the way questions are phrased. One way of trying to ensure that the client does not become disorientated by this process is simply to offer the client explanations both for the need to ask questions in general, as we discussed in the section on closed questions, and for particular questions, especially where these appear not to follow client cues:

> 'Now, at this point, I just need to change the topic for a moment, because I need information about another area to help me understand what you have just said.'

This forms part of the general process of explaining to the client what is happening at each stage in the interview, something to which the same amount of attention should be devoted as to explanation about more physically oriented clinical procedures.

Equally, multiple questions and 'either/or' questions should be avoided, since both serve to disorientate the client. The following is an example of a multiple question:

> 'What happens to you physically; do you get anxious?'

By asking such questions, the interviewer runs into problems both of process and content. Which question is the client to answer? The fact that she is having to think about this issue diverts attention from the interview process, and is therefore possibly damaging to rapport, whilst the quick-fire nature of presenting two ideas together signals that time is tight (whether it is or not), and the qualification of the first question by the second leads the client to a particular type of answer, setting a dangerous precedent for the conduct of the assessment, since the interviewer should seek to convey the impression that it is the client's ideas, rather than her own expectations, that are required. The issue of 'leading the client' also relates to the content of the client's reply, since she is likely to follow this lead, with the result that incorrect or incomplete information may be given. Once again, the client may be unsure as to which part of the question to answer, and may choose one above the other quite arbitrarily, with the other part being ignored. If, as in the above example, an open beginning is followed by a closed qualifying ending, the latter is more likely to be answered. Multiple questions of this kind are little more than verbal habits, and can be easily avoided by thinking for just a few seconds before seeking the question that the interviewer *really* wants answering. In a sense, the point has been rather laboured, since clients are very forgiving of our use of multiple questions, especially if other aspects of the interview are proceeding well, and rapport has been established. There is, however, no reason to make this difficult process more complex than it needs to be.

Either/or questions (e.g. 'Is the problem worse at home or at work?') suffer from broadly the same problems as multiple questions, of which they are a subset. The particular difficulty with such constructions, however, is the range of responses they rule as inadmissible. In the last example, for instance, the true answer might be 'when travelling', yet the client is steered away from such alternatives by the construction of the question. As important as this is the procedural issue, since this indicates both that the interviewer is expecting responses according to her own agenda, and that she has already begun to make up her mind about the nature of the problem. In general, either/or questions also seek to exclude 'middle responses', attempting to dichotomize what are often continuous variables, by encouraging the client to conceptualize the answers in Figure 5.1a rather than 5.1b.

In our earlier discussion of the six Ws, we saw that the question 'why' is sometimes viewed as problematical, since its directness can threaten clients by 'putting them on the spot', in a way reminiscent of schooldays, but I also noted that there might be times when to ask 'why' is of importance. Clearly, if we need to confront someone, for instance about unacceptable behaviour or avoidance of important issues, 'putting them on the spot' is one tactic we might deliberately adopt, and 'why' could be useful here, but it is also important in eliciting and emphasizing the value of the client's views of their difficulties. If we soften the verbal context, as in the following examples:

'I was wondering why . . . '

'Perhaps you'd be the best one to explain why . . . '

'One thing I'm not clear about is why . . . '

rather than:

'Why did you . . . '

'Why have you/haven't you . . . '

we diminish the threatening value of the question by personalizing it, yet retain the directness of style, with its messages about client responsibility and knowledge, and our appreciation and valuing of those attributes. This requires, I believe, a fine touch, and an ability to balance the benefits of offering the client these messages, with the aim of enlisting them as an active partner in intervention, against the possible disruption to the flow of the interview as they attempt to grapple with questions about their motivations and the motivations of others. Such ideas may, as yet, be extremely poorly formed in the client's mind. Indeed, it may be the intervention's precise intention to stimulate consideration of such issues.

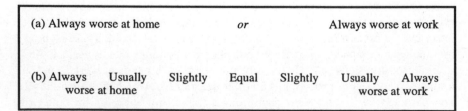

Figure 5.1 Two conceptualizations of client experience

REWARDING CLIENT INFORMATION

This element of cementing the therapeutic contract is more straightforward than the numerous items described under the heading of client orientation. We are all familiar with the operation of rewards in daily life, but these are only rarely recognized as being issues of negotiation between all the participants, possibly because they are often described in the context of studies of animal learning and the teaching and training of children, where power relationships between re-warder and rewarded are often extremely unequal. Nevertheless, cognitive-behavioural assessment (and therapy in general) views reward in a collaborative way, and several writers have written about the reciprocal relationship between participants in a reward setting (e.g. Bandura 1977b; Egan, 1990). Nor is it true to suggest that there is anything mechanical or artificial about reinforcement, unless one also wishes to claim that a good number of our social relationships, starting from the most basic kind, that between mother and infant, are also artificial. Logically, then, whether one makes this claim of artificiality or not, reinforcement is something which is by no means peculiar to intervention settings. It may, however, be used more or less effectively. Interviewers can use reward both to control the flow of client information, in terms of both rate and direction, and to enhance the progress of the therapeutic relationship.

Reinforcement *controls information* from the client by the application of care as to where reinforcing remarks from the interviewer occur. The interviewer who wishes to hear more about a particular topic offers such remarks as:

'Good. I see. OK.'

and demonstrates attention non-verbally when the client pauses (and sometimes during her discourse) and the interviewer wishes her to continue on the same path. If a different direction is indicated, either by client or interviewer, these reinforcing remarks and non-verbal behaviours are offered during the early stages after the change of topic. By this means, the amount of information offered is likely to be increased, and changes of direction smoothed.

Reinforcement *enhances the therapeutic relationship* by demonstrating to the client the interest and approval of the interviewer:

'This seems very important'.

'Thank you for giving such good information/being so honest.'

'I appreciate you helping me with what was quite a long interview'.

It should be emphasized here that such offering of praise to the client is not a sterile piece of manipulation. Good clinicians generally *do* hold positive views about their clients and their capabilities, and clients in turn respond to such views, *when* they are aware of them. Making the client aware of our genuine regard for them is simply a skill to be practised.

REWARDING THE CLIENT'S COPING ABILITIES

In this final element of building a therapeutic relationship during assessment, the notion of expressing our respect for the client is extended into the discussion of their previous attempts at coping with their difficulties. Here, the nurse has two related subgoals: reinforcing *all* client descriptions of previous attempts at coping and selectively reinforcing the content of those attempts which have been most successful, or are most likely to be successful if repeated in the future. Thus, the first subgoal is a reinforcement of the *idea* of coping in general, and aims to boost client confidence, show respect and demonstrate the idea that it is possible to cope with the client's difficulties, thus building hope for the future, whilst the second aims to increase those *specific behaviours* which are likely to lead to continuing success, whilst taking emphasis away from tactics which are likely to prove ineffective. Both subgoals attempt to improve the likelihood of coping behaviours occurring during treatment and beyond. Addressing both these sub-goals is difficult, since the clinician wants to reward coping without rewarding ineffective tactics previously used by the client. In our example of the person with problems of sleeplessness, the nurse will want to reinforce the notion that it is possible to address these difficulties, whilst avoiding rewarding certain tactics, like the use of medication:

> 'Yes, I think discussing the problem with your doctor was a good idea, showing you were starting to think about how to get over the difficulties, but, tell me, could there not be problems with the use of sleeping tablets?'

Also, the client's general approach may need reinforcing, whilst specifics do not:

> 'I find the idea of exercising very impressive as a tactic, and indeed there's a lot of evidence to suggest it might be helpful, but what about the timing of it? Is so soon before going to bed a good idea?'

As an alternative, the interviewer can often simply refrain from commenting about potentially ineffective client coping tactics, and simply concentrate on reinforcing those tactics which are likely to bear fruit. Once again, perhaps because of the roots of reinforcement in behavioural ideas about learning, there is a tendency to think of the above as manipulation of the client. In defence of this, I suggest that here again rewards of this kind are actually quite a normal part of the currency of our daily transactions with each other. The sensitive interviewer merely uses these with more awareness than we might be accustomed to do in daily life. Clients genuinely deserve praise for their attempts at coping with their problems, and equally deserve direction away from those attempts which are unlikely to benefit them.

ORIENTATION OF THE CLIENT TO THE TYPES OF INTERVENTION TO BE OFFERED

We talked in Chapter 4 about this aspect of client orientation, and noted the weakness of the arguments against a full description of intervention, both ethically and practically. In some ways, orientation of the client will occur throughout the course of the nursing relationship, but the assessment interview is an essential starting point, since it is at this juncture that the need for compliance, negotiation and consent begins. A full explanation of treatment should contain at least the following components:

A description of the nurse's initial formulation of the client's difficulties

Clients are often concerned about *what* is wrong with them and *how* this came about, and the skilful interviewer respects this by offering a detailed account of the genesis and maintenance of the problem, where this is possible, or a frank admission that the state of our knowledge does not allow such certainty, along with a series of possible explanations, including their respective likelihoods.

A general description of the rationale underlying the nurse's proposed interventions for the problem

Clearly clients are also concerned about what is to be done regarding their difficulties, but a further goal of rationale-giving is to provide the client with some background to what the nurse will later be attempting to negotiate that she should do in addressing the difficulties, so as to provide a context to help the client remember.

Specific examples of what is likely to be expected of the client

Almost every nursing intervention requires some activity on the part of the client, and the more client-centred approaches obviously require a great deal. For example the use of relaxation exercises in sleeping difficulties requires that the client monitor her sleep pattern, learn and practise the exercises, implement the exercises when sleeplessness occurs, continue to monitor patterns of sleeplessness, and report back accurately on these to the nurse. It may be that the client is unable to carry out the sorts of task the nurse might suggest, or that she feels the degree of handicap caused by the problem does not warrant the investment of time necessitated by such tactics. Although the nurse should strive to be flexible in accommodating the client's personal circumstances, a point is inevitably reached where, if there is no input from the client, no change will occur. Clearly, the client may decide not to proceed with treatment. This is a legitimate decision, for which the client needs adequate information about the specifics of intervention.

Specific examples of what the client can expect of the nurse

Emphasizing the notions of client equality and desire for involvement and negotiation, the nurse makes explicit her commitment to the therapeutic process by explaining her role in the relationship in detail, noting both her specific responsibilities (in the example above, these might include describing self-monitoring, teaching the exercises, helping the client with practice of the exercises, negotiating homework practice, reviewing effectiveness of the exercises) and her more general commitments (e.g. number of proposed sessions, her availability at other times, negotiation of ending of the sessions, contact numbers for use in her absence). The client then has the opportunity to question the appropriateness of these general and specific arrangements.

A prediction about the likelihood of success

Very often, the nurse is endeavouring to help the client by using familiar techniques whose effectiveness has been demonstrated in clients with similar difficulties. The client will want to know what the chances of success are, and needs to know about this both in order to make an informed choice about whether to proceed, and in order to know, at a later date, whether or not to cease the therapeutic liaison. In her turn, the nurse needs to be sufficiently familiar with such information (including numerical success rates where available, since clients often find these revealing) to be able to offer the client a reasonable prediction. Where the nurse is working in areas where the research is divided, or where there is no research evidence, because the problem is either unusual or as yet poorly dealt with by clinicians in general, this issue needs airing with the client. Here it is often helpful to attempt to enlist the client as a co-experimenter in a piece of personal research in which both client and clinician attempt to explore the unfamiliar territory of the client's difficulties.

Emphasis on negotiation

As a final aspect of presenting her orientation to treatment, the nurse takes the opportunity to emphasize the importance of the client's right to negotiate and change both the process and goals of intervention, but also declares that she, *the nurse, has rights in the negotiative process*. In so doing, the nurse attempts to focus on the collaborative nature of treatment, but also offers a lead in to the topics of goal-setting, measurement and evaluation, which will follow as part of assessment, since she explains the importance, for both nurse and client, of defining success and monitoring progress towards it during the course of treatment.

It is only at this point, and after it is certain that all the components of rationale-giving have been offered, that the client can reasonably be asked whether she wishes to pursue treatment and be expected to give an informed decision.

General history-taking

Having achieved a reasonable picture of the client's presenting difficulties and the background specific to them, and agreed with the client that she and the nurse can work together, a useful next stage is to attempt to set the client within the context of her life more generally. This general history-taking is carried out first as a screening exercise, offering the client the opportunity to contribute information which, although less focal to her immediate difficulties, may still be either relevant to them, or may be problematic in other ways. The issues raised may be a long way either from the client's reasons for seeking intervention or from the nurse's area of clinical competence, and there is, therefore, a need for the nurse to be aware of alternative sources of intervention for the client. A further reason for collection of general information about the client is that we may gain useful clues about both possible pitfalls during the course of intervention and possible strengths in other areas of the client's life which she can bring to bear on addressing her difficulties. Thus, if we learn that the client has, for example, an overbearing and opinionated father, who gains from having his daughter dependent upon him, we also can recognize that he is a potential saboteur, whilst discovering that the client is herself an experienced teacher tells us a great deal about how and where to 'pitch' our discussion of aims and objectives, and examination of the client's personal interests will help in discussing and specifying what she might wish to achieve from treatment. It is important to recognize that, even though it is not *focal* to the client's difficulties, general history-taking is never irrelevant. Nor is it an exercise in prying into someone's life – a 'fishing trip' in which we hope that something important may rise to the surface. It should, therefore be governed by the same 'need to know' basis as the rest of our discourse with the client. We aim to find out as much about them as we can, in order to intervene, but no more, in order to avoid violating their privacy. Enough years have passed for me to recount, without breaking confidentiality, a brief episode during a short course I ran on interviewing skills. Whilst I was seeking feedback on the day's events, one participant said of his interview with a role-played client:

'Yes, I got all the information which seemed necessary, but I didn't feel it told me anything interesting.'

Whilst it is a personal regret that I failed on this occasion to transmit to that participant that *anything* a client says is potentially interesting, because of their uniqueness, this remark does demonstrate the difficulty in entering into history-taking with expectations that clients live fascinating lives from which items of purely *biographical* interest will emerge! We need to provide the focus to history-taking by means of the structure we bring to it. One way of doing this is to offer questions which reflect some kind of continuity, helping the client make links between experiences, and therefore increasing the chances of the emergence of rich and relevant material. One method is to begin with a general examination of other areas of the client's life, perhaps starting with inquiry about other areas of difficulty, thus easing the client from the problematic to the less problematic, whilst another is the life-cycle approach in which the client begins with a description of their parents, family and birth circumstances, moving coherently to the present day, and thus to a return to the presenting problems which we will address during goal-setting. Both these suggested approaches have flaws. The first leaves a break in continuity before approaching goal-setting, if this is to be done during the same session, whilst the life cycle approach offers a similar unnatural jump at the beginning, moving the client abruptly away from the here-and-now of her difficulties. Nevertheless, these difficulties in continuity are tolerated well if the nurse introduces the change in emphasis appropriately, as in our earlier description of redirecting the client. The issue is to maintain *some* underlying structure which helps to orient the client and, hopefully, has some congruence with the way she views the world.

GOAL-SETTING AND PLANNING

Many forms of intervention, especially psychological therapies, stress the importance of the nurse–client relationship and of the process of therapy. Given the focus of this book, it is clear that cognitive-behavioural approaches to interviewing also stress these factors. However, what distinguishes the latter from many other approaches is the emphasis on *outcome* and the possibility of quantifying that outcome. One consequence of this emphasis is the precision in interviewing which we have examined throughout the last two chapters, and which finds its most extreme expression in the negotiation with the client of goals of treatment. Gerrard Egan (1990) has asked:

'What difference does it make if clients leave helping sessions with smiles on their faces and songs in their hearts if their problems are not managed more effectively?'

To me, this is a question about the difference between expert process management and expert outcome management, and about the need to quantify the latter. Very little will happen in terms of outcome unless the process of interviewing is managed adequately, and that is why this book concentrates so heavily on process. Nevertheless, all the skilled processing of client information in the world will not help unless the client's behaviour, thoughts and feelings undergo change as a result. In part this relates, it is true, to the selection of appropriate interviewing process tactics which allow decision-making, but the selection of appropriate intervention tactics which the client can employ is crucial. Goal-setting is itself one such tactic, since it represents a way of clarifying often complex client difficulties and helping the client to commit to change, but is also a way of stipulating the criteria a client and clinician should use to decide when desired change has occurred in a given situation. Thus, goal-setting is both therapeutic and evaluative.

Cognitive-behavioural approaches to goal-setting have set a number of indicators of effective specification of desired changes. In part these are derived from the need for precision inherent in the systematic, experimental approach to human behaviour embodied in psychological research. As nurses, we can gain from the approaches of the behaviourist movement in therapy (Shapiro, 1961a; Yule & Hemsley, 1977) and in education (Reilly, 1975), both of which have examined the nature of goal-setting in some detail. The rest of this section represents a consensus of the conclusions reached by these two approaches.

AIMS AND GOALS

We encountered the notions of aims and objectives during our discussion of assessment interviewing in general, and indeed the planning and setting of goals formed one of our aims of assessment. Goal-setting itself, is, in fact, all about specifying and negotiating aims and objectives for treatment. Educationalists have generally regarded aims as general statements of teacher intent. For the nurse, the setting of such personal aims and their sharing with the client may help to focus the progress of intervention, but they should, in the main, be negotiated aims, seeking client agreement at every stage:

> 'Now that we have a good idea of your difficulties, what I was *hoping* to be able to offer would be a series of relaxation exercises.'

In the educationalists' sense, then, aims are what the nurse intends to achieve in terms of what she will offer the client. No improvement by the client is stipulated at this stage as part of the evaluation strategy. The evaluation of whether a nurse's aims have been met is an evaluation of what *quality of care* has been delivered, regardless of its effectiveness. Although this is of rather less interest to the client than actual improvement, its importance lies in the fact that it offers the nurse a strategy through which to judge whether certain baseline performance criteria have been met. The nurse has stated her aims explicitly, and can, therefore, judge whether, for instance, she did in fact meet with the client at the times stated, for the frequency and duration stated, addressing the issues stated in the aim statement. These kinds of aims, sometimes recorded as nursing goals, are quite familiar in nursing care plans using the nursing process, and will not be dwelt on here. Although they are a valid attempt at care assurance, they are not necessarily concerned with client outcome.

CLIENT GOALS AND OBJECTIVES

Although the words 'goal' and 'objective' are used in various ways in the literature, they consistently contain the notions of more and less general pieces of client behaviour change respectively, and it is in this sense that they will be used here. Goals, therefore, represent fairly general statements of what the client might expect to achieve by the end of treatment, whilst objectives are more specific subcomponents of such goals. Additionally, interim objectives may be set by client and clinician to be achieved by particular points during the course of an intervention, and might be taken to represent evidence that the intervention was 'on target'. For the sake of brevity, I shall generally refer to all three outcomes as targets, in Marks's sense of being targeted behaviours, although, in fact, goal statements may well contain a great number of desired changes which are not explicitly stated, and therefore not explicitly targeted. Both goals and objectives should possess the following characteristics in order to be optimally useful in helping client and nurse to assess continuing client achievement.

Goals and objectives should represent a *change desired by the client*. In this sense, the targets need to be connected to the client's handicaps, and represent something which the client would wish to do if she were able. Although this appears obvious, two points are important. Firstly, clients are aware of and influenced by the other people's desire for them to change. As a result, they may give examples of targets which they know the nurse or a relative would like or expect them to meet. To a degree, this is fair enough, and no different from a good many negotiations into which we enter in life away from the treatment setting. The difficulty arises when the client accedes to the goals of another to the detriment of their own wishes, leading to a diminution of their *ownership* of the targets and, therefore, of treatment itself. The ENB managing change documents (ENB, 1989) draw on this notion of ownership and its effect on performance in great detail with regard to initiating change in institutions, and its importance is no less in the case of individual treatment. In consequence, the sensitive nurse questions the client closely about the desirability of a particular stated target, attempting to discover how important that target is to the client, and, therefore, how likely they are to put their best efforts into achieving it.

A second factor is that clients make decisions about targets on the basis of their current experiences of disability. Therefore, a client suffering from long-term pain, when asked whether she wishes to work in the garden each weekend may, not unreasonably, answer 'No', since she perceives this to mean that she must do so in the presence of her current level of pain. If the nurse is lucky, the client may follow this up with: 'it would be too painful' – thus explaining the source of the misunderstanding; if not, the search for client targets may go on, missing, in fact, a highly desired and desirable target. The issue here is that the nurse needs to recognize the client's current perception of her capabilities and exercise care to make explicit the idea that these are targets which the client *would wish* to be able to perform if treatment were to be successful.

This need for explicit language in helping the client to set targets is further illustrated in the requirement that targets represent a *significant change* in the client's well-being. As well as avoiding deflecting the client from desired targets by failing to specify that performance of such behaviours would be contingent upon successful treatment, the nurse also needs to ensure that the client is not herself coming from a position of thinking that little change is possible, and therefore setting her sights too low. Thus, whilst being desired by the client, targets should also actually be likely to make real differences to the way she lives her life. Once again it is important for the nurse to draw the client into a debate about how much change is possible, remembering that the client may have been coping with her difficulties for a considerable time, and, therefore, both have adapted her life considerably to it and have limited ability to look at her future other than in terms of the handicaps caused by her difficulties. Thus, in negotiating targets, part of the role of the nurse is to *offer samples* of what life might be like after successful treatment, and encourage the client to negotiate targets accordingly, so that the client does not set targets which, although achievable (perhaps too easily so) have less effect on her life than targets which she would have liked to achieve but did not dare to think possible.

In contrast, the nurse also needs to guide the client away from setting targets which are *never* going to be achieved. Such suggested outcomes are not only demoralizing for both client and nurse, as both work away to some idealized state of wellness, but are also destructive in that they can conceal a great deal of real change, by wrongly labelling only the idealized end-state as the 'goal'. Principally, two difficulties need to be avoided here. The nurse needs to be aware that whilst many clients may have idealized and stylized memories of what being healthy was like before their difficulties started, with consequent desires to return to this mythical state and the safety it represents, the nurse herself, like all of us, desires to help and cooperate with the client, and is, therefore, in danger of failing to negotiate the client away from these idealized targets, which may also represent the nurse's own desires for perfection, both in her own health and as a clinician. Ellis's list of irrational beliefs of therapists (1983) may be helpful here. This describes some of the irrational beliefs of perfect performance which therapists collect. For example, therapists (including nurses) may believe that they must succeed with all clients, or be more successful than other therapists. At the end of this chapter, I ask you to read Ellis's article, and perform an exercise based upon it. When you have examined the article, I strongly advise that you add one other negative thought to the list: 'Assuming that I should never have any of the thoughts on this list' – for this is itself an irrational assumption.

Having described the problem of idealized assumptions about what health is like, and therefore about the nature of improvement, it must also be noted that the nurse can give mistaken impressions to the client about what is practically possible during treatment. Thus, the need for the nurse to give as accurate an account as possible about likely outcomes, which we encountered in the section on orientation of the client to the therapeutic approach, is important again in the context of target-setting, when the nurse should guide the client towards an understanding of what outcomes are practicable given the length, scope and focus of intervention. Client targets should, therefore, be *practically achievable* within the constraints of time and resources.

Since it is impossible to be exhaustive in stipulating *all* the complexities of a client's experiences (or even simply her difficulties), not every behaviour can be targeted, with the result that the nurse attempts to make those targets which are explicitly stated not only valuable in themselves to the client, but also *representative of improvements in other areas* of difficulty which are not so stated. For example, it is reasonable to expect, from our last example, that improvement on a target such as 'To work in my garden at weekend, bending to do the weeding' would also represent improvement in bending over for other activities (retrieving dropped items, rising from a low chair, etc.). We *could* go through and specifically target each such behaviour separately, and we might indeed do so less formally as part of interim target-setting during the course of treatment, but to make each separate instance of essentially similar difficulties a separate summative objective is unwieldy and often redundant, given the principle of generalization of learning across similar situations. A good general rule is: the more similar the events, the fewer the number of targets.

All the above issues are open to negotiation, which the nurse offers as part of the target-setting exercise, again offering an experience in brief of the collaborative nature of intervention. In this way, targets become the joint public property of client and nurse, representing a contract of care in which each partner has duties, and a statement of commitment to change from both partners, reflecting their initial negotiations. We now turn to an examination of the components of each target statement.

In order to render them sufficiently specific to allow us to estimate client success during an intervention, targets should state what the desired behaviour is, the *frequency* with which it is desired that a given activity be performed, the *duration* for which it is desired that it be performed, the *setting* in which it is to be performed and any *additional criteria* which would indicate its successful performance. In helping the client to investigate and specify targets, the nurse many benefit from the use of the six Ws, inquiring what the client wishes to be able to, when, where and who with she wishes to do it, what she requires others to, and why she wishes to be able to do it. Once again, it is worth noting that asking such questions need not be undertaken in the didactic way I have presented them here. Let's return to our example of the client who wished to be able to tolerate working in her garden, and examine a sample target for her.

> *Target 1*: To be able to weed my garden, involving bending over (desired activity and setting), every Saturday and Sunday (frequency) for one hour on each occasion (duration), without help from others, without medication, and with no more than 20% of my current resting pain (additional criteria for success).

This represents a real enhancement of the person's life, and, to be an important target, would, necessarily, be of considerable difficulty before treatment is commenced. Therefore, the interim targets we mentioned earlier will be important stepping stones for client and nurse in working towards the end-point target. We shall return to this topic in Chapter 7, but for the present, here are some sample interim targets, informally agreed by client and nurse for various stages during intervention.

> Practise relaxation exercises on five occasions this week.
> Practise altering posture exercises from sitting to standing position on 10 occasions daily.
> Weed in the garden for 20 minutes on one occasion this week, whilst maintaining attention to all alterations of posture.
> Record all instances of 'guarding' my back by tensing muscles, and follow each episode with 2 minutes relaxation of those muscles.

In this example, you will note that there are no instances of others helping the client perform her practice routines. Nor are any others involved in her progress through actual subgoals of treatment. In other cases, early subgoals and exercise regimes may well need the supervision, aid and interventions of others. This will be particularly true of both the acutely ill client, and the client who requires a great deal of guidance through a complicated set of interventions for complex difficulties. Although the eventual goal is client independence, target statements should acknowledge that this goal is not always achievable early in an intervention (or in some cases, ever).

MEASUREMENT

Target-setting implies the idea of measurement of the level of severity of the client's difficulties and, hopefully, the quantitative monitoring of the diminution of that severity. However, Kirk (1989) has noted that this monitoring has often been done informally. She also describes Shapiro's (1961b) characterization of behavioural interventions as including the application of scientific method to the evaluation of client distress, and a number of advantages associated with the use of this method. The nursing process in general also benefits from this scientific approach, although formal numerical measurement of client difficulties as a routine part of nursing interventions is a comparatively rare feature of the nursing literature.

Kirk suggests that measurement is advantageous for four main reasons. First, it allows greater accuracy in the description of the problem than does free retrospective evaluation by the client. Second, it allows greater scope for modification of the intervention programme in the light of feedback. Third, the act of measurement can itself be therapeutic, for example by helping the client to calibrate her experiences against her personal 'bests' and 'worsts'. This can be particularly important in helping to generate hope and confidence in clients who have been experiencing difficulty for an extended period of time. Finally, measurement helps the nurse to establish whether the interventions negotiated with the client have, in fact, been carried out as agreed, with regard both to frequency and content. In cognitive-behavioural assessment, then, as we noted earlier, target-setting provides an initial chance for the nurse to introduce the client to the notion of measurement of her difficulties, by guiding her through measurement of the targets they have agreed and any formal measures associated with such targets. Since the concept of measurement may be quite new to the client, it is important that sufficient time is devoted both to the process itself, and to an explanation of its relevance:

'Now that we have agreed these targets together, I'm going to suggest that we try and actually measure them, in some numerical way, so we can check how treatment is going, and, hopefully, get some feedback on your progress as the days go by. It will also help us to consider changes we might wish to make if it turns out that things are not going as well as we might have wished.'

This is a good general introduction, and the nurse could continue with:

'Here are some forms that I use quite a lot, and, as you can see, I've used them to write down your targets, as we discussed together just now.'

or:

'Are there any measurements you are used to using in your line of work which we could adapt to help us with using measurement in looking at your difficulties?'

The second example has the advantage of helping the client to come to an ownership of the conceptual framework she and the nurse will be using. In research, this amount of freedom can lead to difficulties in drawing comparisons between one client's response and another's, but, in clinical practice, the flexible nurse may well find this problem outweighed by the therapeutic usefulness of greater client involvement and decision-making. Figure 5.2 illustrates one target-setting measure, based on a 'visual analogue scale' (e.g. Karoly, 1985). Additionally, measures can often be borrowed from the work of other nurses, doctors and psychologists, and the sections on further reading in this book contain a number of texts where the authors use such formal measures. Perhaps the best way to understand about measurement is to follow the exercise given at the end of this chapter.

TARGETS

1:

Please make a mark on the line below in the place which best illustrates your response to the following statement:

My progress towards achieving this target regularly without difficulty

0%   100%

2:

Please make a mark on the line below in the place which best illustrates your response to the following statement:

My progress towards achieving this target regularly without difficulty

0%   100%

3:

Please make a mark on the line below in the place which best illustrates your response to the following statement:

My progress towards achieving this target regularly without difficulty

0%   100%

Figure 5.2 A target-setting measure

Taken together, these last two elements – goal-setting and measurement – complete the bulk of baseline information-gathering. The characteristics of effective goal-setting and measurement are summarized in Figure 5.3. We now turn to the issue of closure of the assessment session.

Throughout this chapter, we have stressed the need for reinforcement of client efforts at coping, including the transmission to the nurse of accurate information. At the end of the session, the nurse has the chance to offer *final reinforcement*, and this is a major component of interview closure. Reinforcement of client efforts is particularly important following the assessment interview, since, at this point, the client has only begun to engage in treatment. This beginning commitment may well be a source of some disquiet for the client, and the interviewer attempts, therefore, both to acknowledge the degree of courage the client has shown in committing to examination of her difficulties, and to ensure that hope with regard to the future is also offered. With regard to the latter, if the earlier stages of the interview have been handled appropriately, the client already has some reason to be optimistic about the progress of treatment, since she has seen the nurse's interest in her difficulties, and expertise in handling the interview situation and explaining what intervention will involve. In the final stages of the interview, the nurse adds to this by entering into early negotiations with the client both about future appointments, thus stressing the idea of continuity, and about what the client may do between the current session and the next. In our examin-

---

Effective targets should be:

    Desired by the client
    Expressive of significant change
    Practically achievable
    Representative of other changes

Effective targets should state:

    The target behaviour
    Its frequency
    Its duration
    Its setting
    Its criteria

Effective measures should:

    Be negotiated with the client
    Reflect the target behaviours precisely
    Be frequent
    Allow accurate specification of problems
    Allow modification of treatment
    Allow calibration by the client
    Allow monitoring of client performance

Figure 5.3 Effective baseline measurement

ation of education of the client in Chapter 6 we will examine this setting of interim targets in much more detail. At this stage, it suffices to note that it is intended, in the context of the assessment interview, to (a) focus primarily on the collection of more baseline information, where necessary, (b) give the client an early taste of the collaborative nature of intervention and (c) give the client an early taste of success in following negotiated therapeutic instructions. Thus, homework tasks at this stage should be simple and easily within the client's reach. As part of the negotiations, the interviewer also clarifies what she herself will be doing with regard to the client's difficulties between sessions.

At this point in the interview, the interviewer can elicit from the client *final feedback* about the progress of the interview, attempting to find out what her own performance was like, whether the interview has met client expectations, and whether the client has final questions and comments. *Closing summaries* by the interviewer regarding the whole of the interview can, as well as giving the client final evidence of the interviewer's interest, help to set the scene for such client questions. Figure 5.4 offers a template which can be used for closing most interviews. The issue of allowing time for anxiety reduction to occur is rarely a factor during assessment interviews, and so is discussed in detail in Chapter 7.

Final reinforcement

Negotiation of next steps in treatment

Practical arrangements (appointments, letters)

Final feedback from client

Final summaries from interviewer

Final questions from client

(Allowing time for anxiety reduction to occur)

Figure 5.4 Interview closure

CLINICAL EXAMPLE

The case material which follows explores both these issues and the whole of the assessment process from the viewpoint of an interview with a client, Mr Weems, suffering from asthma, who has been referred to Jane, the nurse, by his GP, for help in managing his inhaler medication, which has become out of control. We will leave other aspects of his difficulty to emerge during the course of the interview. You are reminded, however, that many of the client's responses will be considerably truncated, since the main focus of this text is upon *interviewer* behaviour. For the purposes of this example, we will assume that the opening material dealt with in Chapter 2 has already been covered when we join the interview:

Jane: So, perhaps you could start by telling me, in general terms, about the issues which have brought you here today? (*General open question.*)

Mr W: Well, it's about my inhaler. The doctor says I'm using far too much of it.

Jane: What do you think yourself? (*Keeping focus on need to see client's idea of the difficulty, although a pause would be equally good here.*)

Mr W: I know well enough that the amount I'm using has increased just of late, but I can't seem to slow down on using it.

Jane: It sounds like *controlling it* is the problem. (*Following the cue in Mr Weems's statement.*)

Mr W: Definitely. Every time I go anywhere, I have to have it with me just in case!

Jane: What might happen if you didn't have it with you? (*Specific open question aiming to elicit maintaining factors in Mr Weems's problem.*)

Mr W: Well, I worry that I'll have an attack, and that I won't be able to do anything about it.

Jane: OK. Now you've told me so far that there is difficulty with the use of your inhaler, which you reckon you've increased the use of, and mentioned in particular what happens when you're out. (*Summarizing.*) I want now to ask you in a bit more detail about what happens when you use the inhaler, focussing on what happens when you're out to start with, and also looking at what you've called the attacks. (*Orientation of the client to the material to follow.*) Will that be OK? (*Initial seeking of client consent/negotiation.*)

Mr W: Sure. I must say, though, that I don't go out that much, just at present.

Jane: OK, thank you for telling me that (*Reinforcement of offer of information and transmission of respect to the client*), and we'll look at that in detail later. For the moment, let me just ask you first of all (*Redirecting the client*) to run through the situations where you use the inhaler. (*Starting on the six Ws to identify the precise problematic behaviours.*)

Mr W: Well, anywhere, really, if I think I'm going to have an attack. (*Antecedent information.*) Usually away from home, though – especially if its a long way away. Driving can be quite difficult.

Jane: Give me an example of what might happen when you're driving.

Mr W: I often start to get a tightness in my chest, and if it gets any worse and I start to get wheezy, then I'd take a couple of puffs.

Jane: So, there would be some tightness and wheezing. Any other physical feelings? (*Eliciting autonomic/physical information about antecedents to the proposed problematic episode 'use of the inhaler'.*)

Mr W: Quite often I feel sweaty, and my heart thumping in my chest . . .

Jane: And that would make you say certain things to yourself? (*Question about cognitions, but phrased as a statement.*)

Mr W: Yes, it's very frightening.

Jane: It certainly sounds like it is. (*Validating client's perception and showing respect.*) I wonder if it might make you think any particular things (*Still chasing the cognition – looking for specifics.*)

Mr W: Yes, that I might choke, or faint, or even that I might die.

   (Jane pauses, nods and leans forward.)

Jane: That's the main fear.

   (Mr W nods.)

Jane: And what do you do then? (*Eliciting behaviour.*)

Mr W: Then I'd use the inhaler.

Jane: 'A couple of puffs', I think you said earlier – is that right? (*Eliciting frequency.*)

Mr W: Usually.

Jane: Usually? (*Encouraging specificity.*)

Mr W: Sometimes, it might be three puffs, or I might wait a minute and then take another two.

Jane: Thank you. It's very important to get as exact a picture as possible. (*Rewarding information without rewarding the problematic attempt at coping.*) Is there anything else you do during these episodes?

   Here Jane goes on to examine other aspects of the client's behaviours when he requires medication. She might, for example, find that he ceases activity, asks for reassurance from those around, sits down. There may also be positive attempts at coping.

Mr W: Sometimes I used to try and wait for a while before taking the inhaler, to see if the breathlessness would pass.

Jane: Excellent. That seems like a good tactic, though I guess it can be very difficult sometimes, when you're worried about what will happen. (*Rewarding attempts at coping.*) Can we move on to look at what happens next – after you've used the inhaler.

Mr W: I generally feel a lot calmer then. Even when I open the inhaler, I'm already starting to think 'This'll make it all right'.

Jane: Even before you take it. (*Letting the client see the significance of his words.*) And the thoughts you have afterwards? (*Returning to the topic of cognitions about consequences of the problematic behaviours.*)

Jane then goes on to ask about the physical features which follow the episode, and about Mr Weems's activity at this time. Throughout the above brief examination of a single episode, Jane does not mechanically run through a fixed protocol, but follows what Mr Weems wants to discuss in the first instance, tailoring it to her interviewing style, and only occasionally redirecting to keep focus. Hence, if Mr Weems begins with a description of cognitions, Jane follows this, then completes the three systems by asking about behaviour and autonomic/physical effects. Similarly, she does not, at the beginning of the interview, launch into a nurse-led examination of the three systems, but follows Mr Weems's description of an incident by asking for more behavioural detail about it (starting the six Ws), prior to redirection to the ABC.

At this point in the interview, Jane could continue by examining other instances of the problematic behaviours, using the ABC model as before, and rounding out the picture of the client by means of (S)pecifiers. Here is how Jane applies specifiers to inhaler use during car driving.)

Jane: Now you've described using the inhaler when driving, and told me that roughly the same kinds of thoughts and feelings apply as when you're out walking, but with the additional worry that you might crash the car and injure people. We've also noted that you use the inhaler in the car much more than at other times. Is that right? (*Summarizing and seeking feedback about content.*)

Mr W: (Nods)

Jane: I believe I now need even more specific information about your difficulty when driving. Can you see how that will help me to clarify my picture of your problem? (*Seeking feedback about the appropriateness of an aspect of the agenda.*)

Mr W: Yes, I can see you need an understanding of it all before you can know if you can help.

Jane: Thank you. Can we now try and get even more specific about what happens at these times. Hopefully this will also help us build up a picture of the effect of the problem on your life. (*Orientating the client as to the purpose of a line of questioning.*) Firstly, how often do you use the inhaler on an average journey? (*Frequency – closed question.*)

Mr W: Mostly I drive into town – that takes about 20 minutes each way. I could use the inhaler three or four times altogether.

Jane: And you'd do that journey how often? (*Closed question to clinch detail about frequency.*)

Mr W: Every day.

Jane: OK, thanks. Now I wonder if it makes a difference who is with you on these journeys?

Mr W: Definitely. If the kids are in the car, I tend to take the inhaler more. Especially if they're fooling around.

Jane: So there is something about them being there that makes you more likely to use the inhaler. *This is really a rephrasing of the question 'Why do you use the inhaler more when they are present' as a statement.*

Mr W: There are a couple of things, I suppose. I worry that things might happen to them if I had an attack, but also, if they're fooling about I find it difficult to concentrate on the driving, as well.

Jane: What do people do if they see you using the inhaler in the car?

Mr W: It depends. If it's the kids, they often don't notice. If they do, they'll say 'Are you all right, Daddy?', or something. If it's my wife, she usually asks if I'm OK, but she also often gets annoyed if I've used it a lot that day.

Jane: What does that make you feel? (*Looking for more information about how the problem and the reactions of others interact.*)

Mr W: Funnily enough, that's actually quite reassuring – it's like if Mary's angry with me then there's no problem. You know, nothing to worry about.

Jane: Yes, I know what you mean. It's as though you know she wouldn't be annoyed if she felt that you were in danger. Apart from having other people about, are there any other things that we haven't touched on that make the problem better or worse?

          So far, Jane has asked (S)pecifier questions about the problematic episodes. She now goes on to ask specifiers about the problem as a whole.

Jane: Now you told me earlier that you've had asthma for many years – 20, I think you said. When did you first notice you were using more of the inhaler than seemed reasonable?

          This question about onset may be followed up by a series of ABC questions about circumstances surrounding onset, where these can be remembered by the client.

Jane: Have there been any times when the use of the inhaler has been significantly more or less than usual?

Jane: Have you any ideas yourself about what is maintaining your increased use of the inhaler?

Although to continue in this way would demand a whole further chapter, just to transcribe eliciting the presenting problem, you can begin to see how Jane builds up her picture of the client's difficulties. In the following interchanges, she continues her orientation of the client by explaining both her formulation of his difficulties, and the rationale for the steps she will propose they take together in addressing them.

Jane: Now, *I* think I have all the information I need for now. Are there any particular issues which I *should* have asked you about or you didn't feel *you* had the chance to tell me about in sufficient detail?

Mr W: No, I don't think so.

Jane: Well, at this stage, I'd like to thank you again for giving me such good information. It's certainly been helpful. (*Reinforcement.*) I'd like now to try and give you an idea of what I think is going on here, and then, with your permission, explain a bit about how I feel we might work together. (*Further orientation.*) There will also be time to ask me questions as we go along, and again at the end (*Stressing the need for understanding, interaction and negotiation.*)

You mentioned earlier that you thought a lot of the difficulty was to do with anxiety, and I certainly agree with that. Let's look at how that might work in practice, taking the example of the car. It seems that you become aware of the beginning of some unpleasant physical sensations, like tightening of the chest, which you have associated with the start of asthma attacks in the past. That makes you feel anxious, so you add to the difficulty by thinking anxiety-provoking thoughts, and your physical symptoms start to increase as you get the physical symptoms of anxiety on top. Since these symptoms are quite similar, in some ways, to what happens in asthma attacks, they seem like further evidence that an attack is about to happen, so the frightening thoughts get stronger, and you take the inhaler, even though you would prefer not to, but to wait and see. Taking the inhaler helps, of course, and not only because of helping with your breathing. It also reassures you that things will be all right, and you have come to associate the two events – taking the inhaler and decreased anxiety – just as I might associate sitting in my favourite armchair at the end of the day with feeling relaxed. Now it is quite likely, given that we have not been able to identify any physical triggers, that increased use of the inhaler has, in fact, *increased* the problem, since you never get to cope with the anxiety associated with the *possibility* of an attack by yourself, without medication. *General formulation of problem according to a cognitive-behavioural viewpoint.*

Well, I have said a lot, and I wonder what you think about it? (*Seeking feedback about the 'fit' of her perceptions of the problem with the client's.*)

Mr W: I did expect you to say something of the sort. I do realize that I've become dependent on it in a way I never used to be, and I think I understand about how that's happened.

Jane: Good. Can you, for my benefit, and so I know I've explained it right, feed back to me what I said about the likely cause of the problem?

Mr W: Yes. (*Feeds back.*)

Jane: As regards treatment, in general, this sort of difficulty is best helped by gradual reduction of the medication, which it is thought comes to be overused because of its role in rewarding you by decreasing anxiety, and by learning different ways of coping with the fear that the possibility of attacks gives rise to. Reduction of anxiety happens primarily because you learn *through direct experience* that the attacks do not, in fact, always occur if you don't take the inhaler, and that anxiety goes away on its own. (*General rationale for intervention.*) I'm sure that in your life there have been things that you have been anxious about that you've *had* to face, and that the anxiety has gone down in time.

Mr W: Yes, I was involved in a rail crash about 12 years ago – just a minor one – and I felt very worried about travelling on trains, but I couldn't stop using the train, and very quickly, I stopped even thinking about the dangers.

Jane: That's exactly what I mean! That's also what treatment would be about. For instance, we might agree that you would go out with the inhaler in the glove compartment in the car, and not take it out until a certain amount of time had passed after the first signs of an attack. Then we might gradually lengthen the time between these two events – onset of an episode and use of the inhaler. At the same time, I would ask you to do a number of exercises to help you cope with the very real fears this would arouse. For instance, we might learn relaxation exercises, and also practise a series of coping thoughts you could say to yourself instead of the frightening thoughts we've identified during this conversation. (*Specific description of likely treatment tactics the client would be required to carry out.*)

Mr W: So I'd be learning to do without the inhaler?

Jane: We would do everything we could, in a sense, to give you the experience of coping with the anxiety associated with the onset of an attack without using the inhaler. This would help you discriminate between feelings which are or are not likely to lead on to a full blown asthma episode, but would be difficult and possibly frightening in the first place. However, we would work as a team, organizing exactly how the treatment would be scheduled between the two of us. (*Emphasis on negotiation.*) My part in the proceedings apart from teaching you the exercises I mentioned, would be to help you to monitor progress, negotiate with you the sorts of tasks you could be doing to help in addressing the problem, and generally support you through what could be a potentially difficult time. (*Explicit description of the role of the nurse.*) In a lot of ways, you would be becoming your own therapist, and you would have a more and more active role in deciding treatment as we went on. (*Emphasis on collaboration.*)

Thinking now about the effectiveness of this way of proceeding, I can tell you that there is a certain amount of evidence that it is useful in dealing with the difficulties you describe. Certainly there is a great deal to suggest that, in terms of dealing with anxiety *in general*, it is the best course of action, and that the success rate is at least 70 per cent, looking at anxiety problems as a whole. Since your own difficulty is comparatively unusual, I can't give you quite that kind of assurance, but I can guarantee you that we will examine closely how treatment is going at every stage. I myself have dealt with difficulties similar to you own on a number of occasions, and all those people were able to substantially reduce their medication use. (*As well as offering an estimate of outcome, and introducing the need for evaluation for the first time, Jane also presents the client with images of her own success (demonstrating relevant expertise) and that of other clients in positions similar to that of Mr Weems, offering them as positive models for him.*)

Here Jane would again invite questions and recaps from the client, to elicit his understanding of the rationale she has presented, and seek his formal consent to begin the intervention. The above is a 'bare bones' approach to rationale giving, and many cognitive-behaviourists would stress the need for commitment from the client, the importance of long periods of time spent in the anxiety-provoking situations, the need for the involvement of family and friends as allies in treatment. Whether this occurs during an initial assessment, or later during treatment negotiation is a matter for debate. Similarly, nurses familiar with other traditions would stress other aspects of the problem, for example going into great detail about the nature of physiological changes during anxiety and describing the conduct of relaxation exercises in equal detail. What is presented here is a general template for rationale-giving.

After general history-taking, Jane goes on to set targets with the client, and introduce the concept of measurement, guiding the client through a series of measures relevant to his difficulties.

Jane: Now that we have more or less completed this information-gathering part of treatment, and before we begin to talk about specific things which might be helpful in coping with the difficulty with increased inhaler use, we will go on to identify some targets which you would hope to achieve by the end of treatment. This will give us both something to work towards.

Mr W: Is that like the goals we spoke about when you asking how the problem affects my life?

Jane: Yes. I hope we'll be able to identify a series of things you can't do now, because of the problem, but that you would wish to do. It's more than that, though, because I'm going to be asking you to be *very specific* about what it is that you want to achieve, and we'll write it down so we can look back on it later in treatment. Then we'll know if what we're doing is on the right track, and we'll be able to decide about making alterations if we need to. Is there anything which springs to mind immediately.

Mr W: Well, the obvious thing is to decrease using the inhaler.

Jane: Yes. What sort of amount of inhaler use seems reasonable to you?

Mr W: Well, I'm thinking back to when I was just using it like the doctor told me – before I had the problem, I mean. Then it seemed to be about two or three times a day.

Jane: And that was sufficient for you?

Mr W: Well, nine times out of ten, yes.

Jane: Fine. I've written that down like this, as a start: 'To use my inhaler no more than three times a day.' Would that be two puffs each time?

Mr W: Yes, but what if I need to use it more?

Jane: Well, did you before you had the problem?

Mr W: Very occasionally.

Jane: Could you give me a rough estimate? (*Encouraging the client to specify.*)

Mr W: Say once a month.

Jane: OK. It's your target, so let's incorporate that last bit into it. It could read: 'To use my inhaler (two puffs each time) no more than three times a day, on 90 per cent of occasions'. That '90 per cent' part is to take into account for the odd times when you might need to use it more – maybe because of weather conditions, or exertion – as you did in the past. Is that more reasonable, now?

Mr W: Yes, but I just wonder how I'm ever going to achieve it.

Jane: Sure. I appreciate that it seems like a heck of a mountain to climb at present. Remember, though, that this is a target for the *end* of treatment, not for tomorrow or the day after. It's something to be worked gradually towards.

(*Pause.*)

Jane: Now, at this stage I hope that we can start to measure the difficulty of your target. It's quite important that you mentioned how difficult it seemed, and measuring is one way of us getting feedback on your improvement as we go through with treatment. This seems to be a more accurate way than just talking informally. I've written your target out on this form, which is one I use quite often. (*Shows Figure 5.5*) As you can see, there's a line below your target statement, and at one end there's written '100 per cent', and at the other, 'zero per cent'. I want to ask you to make a mark on that line which corresponds to how much success you've had so far in achieving what we have written down as a target – to give us a basis on which to judge your progress. Don't worry about scoring high – remember this is the very beginning of treatment. (*Jane has a slight problem here – it would have been better to offer this reassurance after the client had recorded his score. Doing so beforehand may well bias the response. Of course, this has to be balanced against clients' tendency to 'score good' on charts which rate success, because of their own desire not to admit the degree of seriousness of the problem.*)

OK, that's fine. If we now measure that line, we can see that you think you've made something like about, oh, 5 per cent progress, even before we start treatment. Is that about what you reckon? (*Seeking validation for the scale and checking the client's understanding of it.*)

TARGETS

1: To use my inhaler (two puffs each time) no more than three times a day, on 90 per cent of occasions

Please make a mark on the line below in the place which best illustrates your response to the following statement:

My progress towards achieving this target regularly without difficulty

0%_____100%

2:

Please make a mark on the line below in the place which best illustrates your response to the following statement:

My progress towards achieving this target regularly without difficulty

0%_____100%

Figure 5.5 Mr Weems's target statement

Mr W: Yes, I think so. I'm thinking of the attempts I've made to hold off on using the inhaler.

Jane: Yes, I thought so. That seems about right. Are there any other ways you can think of we could measure this target of inhaler reduction.

Mr W: Well indirectly, yes. I have to collect quite a few repeat prescriptions! (Smiles.)

Jane: (Nods enthusiastically) Excellent. So we could record the number of times you have to do that over say . . . (pause)

Mr W: Perhaps the next month?

> *Jane can now go on to organize with the client a series of further targets for the end of treatment, taking baseline measures for each one. The general point to notice here is that Mr Weems is encouraged, from the beginning, to take an active role in target-setting, specification and measurement, emphasizing his ownership of the targeting process and of treatment in general.*

UNUSUAL ASSESSMENT SITUATIONS

In some senses, the cognitive-behavioural approach does not accept the value of the distinction between routine and unusual interviews. There are just *interviews*, and these are all approached according to their merits, using the three systems approach and having due regard to the assumptions about the client made in Chapter 1. Nevertheless, it is undoubtedly true that some interviews give interviewers more trouble than others. In this section, we shall briefly examine these interviews, explore what makes them different from the assessment interviews we have already discussed, and offer some ways of attempting to focus on the client in spite of the difficulties associated with the unusual interview. Much of the information which follows is equally applicable to interviews other than assessment, but is included here because it is related to issues of engaging the client in treatment, which characteristically occurs in the early stages of a cycle of interviews, or because it addresses issues which are especially problematic during the early stages, when the client is unfamiliar to the interviewer.

The brief interview

One major characteristic of the brief interview is that it is often *ad hoc* in character. Thus, we may be asked questions by clients or relatives whilst in the middle of some other communication, required to answer some query on the telephone, and so on. Most nurses, particularly those who work in hospital settings, are familiar with the constant interruptions which form part of their normal working day and conspire to break down any continuity of their communication. This seems to immediately break our guideline regarding the need for adequate preparation for the interview and adequate time and attention in carrying it out. However, clients do require a response at the time, and the successful interviewer makes the best use of any situation which is available for client communication and is aware that these chance meetings may be built upon in later, more structured interactions with the interviewee. In order to maximize the benefit to be gained from the brief interview, the interviewer may:

Share her time problem with the client.
Bear in mind aspects of beginning interviews described in Chapter 2 and employ as much of this information as possible in the given time.
Find out what the client's concern is, in brief.
Act accordingly (refer to another staff member, arrange to meet later, offer brief information)
Make a note of what has been agreed, since her attention is likely to be poor.
Adhere precisely to what has been agreed with the client.

The main purpose of these elements of the brief interview is to allow a fuller examination of the client's concerns at some later time. In order to facilitate this later interview as much as possible, the interviewer attempts to demonstrate the positive interviewer characteristics described in earlier chapters, thus reinforcing the client for asking to speak to her and increasing the likelihood that such approaches will be repeated. Thus, even the unprepared interview has goals for the interviewer, which provide a structure to the interaction:

Demonstrate respect for the client.
Address the client's difficulty where possible.
Offer a rationale for declining an interview of appropriate length.
Maximize the likelihood of a productive further meeting

THE GROUP INTERVIEW

This refers to any interview when more than a single interviewee is present, including family, friends and other professionals. To approach the topic of family interviewing or group counselling in any depth at all would require a book in itself. However, some basic guidelines for survival in the group interview are offered, primarily focussing on interviewer behaviour in the information-gathering interview. Five general types of extra demand are made of the interviewer in the group interview: demands of attention, demands of evidence, demands of negotiation, demands of arbitration, demands of time.

The interviewer conducting a group interview will find that a great deal is happening. Not only may several people be trying to give information at once, but they will also be interacting with each other in ways which will very likely be of importance in an examination of the client's (or group's) difficulties. It is well established that humans can learn to attend to a wide array of incoming information and to perform several tasks at once (e.g. Shaffer, 1975), but it is equally well demonstrated that, in the absence of a great deal of practice, performance rapidly declines as the number and complexity of the tasks increases. Thus, group interviews are particularly difficult for the inexperienced, who would be wise to avoid them, perhaps beginning by *interviewing each participant individually, then bringing them together for the final phase of the interview*. This has the additional advantage of allowing each to give their account in confidence. The precise rules of confidentiality which apply in such situations need discussion and agreement with all concerned before commencing. As an additional tactic, the interviewer can enlist a co-interviewer, to help record the progress of the interview, or, with permission, use prosthetic measures such as video and audio tape recording. Finally, the interviewer can allow the presence of all participants, but interview them serially, having negotiated with them the order of contribution.

The problem of evidence arises when the co-interviewees offer conflicting accounts of events. Inevitably, the interviewer has either to make some judgement about which is the correct account, or to lose any value the information might have by refraining to make such a judgement. In this situation, helping the interviewees to come to a consensus about events may resolve this difficulty, although the consensus may itself represent some distortion of the true state of affairs, being vulnerable to bias associated with the relative power of the co-interviewees.

The issue of evidence leads naturally to the problem for the interviewer of being required to be an arbitrator between these conflicting accounts, and also the conflicting feelings of the participants about aspects of their difficulties. In extreme cases, clients may become involved in open argument in front of the interviewer, as each attempts to enlist her allegiance. The *interviewer must avoid this role* except where this has been has been specifically negotiated with all parties as part of the process of the intervention (as in some aspects of cognitive-behavioural family therapy). As alternatives, the interviewer can:

Feed back to the interviewees their behaviour.
Reward aspects of behaviour in the interview which do not involve argument.
Contract with the interviewees that only one will speak at a time, and reinforce information from the speaker and silence from the other participant(s).
Ignore the argumentative behaviour and repeat information-seeking questions (withdrawal of reinforcement)
Stop the interview if it becomes apparent that argumentative behaviour will not cease (withdrawal of reinforcement) and agree to meet again to negotiate an alternative way of proceeding.

I have drawn the distinction between arbitration and negotiation, in that the interviewer is less of an observer and more of a participant in the latter. Whilst the principle of negotiation in treatment s unchanged in the group interview, the interviewer needs to be aware of the necessity of getting the agreement of a number of participants. Thus, particular care is needed in order to ensure that all parties understand the process and content of the negotiations, and equal care is required to guarantee mutual satisfaction.

The final demand, time, springs from the other difficulties noted above. Group interviews often take longer than individual interviews because of the number of additional aspects which have to be taken into account by the interviewer. Thus, the interviewer who is short of time would be unwise to offer group interviews as a way of attempting to save it. Group interviews are offered for the *additional* benefits they confer in terms of increased information and the opportunity to observe the client interacting with others.

THE RELUCTANT CLIENT

We touched on the subject of the reluctant client in our initial discussion of the assumptions made by cognitive-behaviourists about clients. Often, the reluctant client is no different from any other client showing avoidance behaviour. In other words, she is displaying a characteristic human reaction to fearful or other aversive stimuli, and the job of the interviewer is to arrive at an understanding of how those stimuli operate to her detriment in her life. In practical terms, the interviewer needs to accept the client's reluctance as simply another piece of assessment information. Where the reluctance of the client to enter into the interview springs from fear at confronting her difficulties, the interviewer's position is comparatively simple, and involves continuing negotiation with the client of the speed at which the interview will progress, so as to allow her sufficient time to demonstrate that she can cope with each stage of giving information about her difficulties. However, a significant number of reluctant clients do not experience difficulty in engaging in the interview because of anxiety about facing their problems. Whilst it would be pleasant to believe that all clients entered into treatment of their own free will, this is not always so. Whilst the hospitalized anorexic we mentioned in Chapter 1, and other groups of compulsorily treated clients represent one end of the spectrum of reluctant clients, there are many more clients who, whilst not treated compulsorily, are coerced with more or less force by people around them to enter treatment. The claim of Szasz (1960) that clients can enter into treatment as equal partners in a contract is a piece of naive and misplaced libertarianism. In real life, even the self-referred client enters into treatment for many reasons, some of which are responses to the exhortation and bullying of others. Nevertheless, if these people have life problems, are they not equally worthy of intervention? For the interviewer, the problem is where to begin, and we noted in Chapter 1 the importance of finding common ground with the client on which to negotiate. Thus, the imprisoned paedophile may not, prior to treatment, see anything wrong with his practices, and it is therefore meaningless to try to negotiate treatment goals based on the premiss that he does. He may, however, see a great deal wrong with being imprisoned (the aversive stimulus working in *his* life), and this may form the beginning point of an intervention programme. For the interviewer, the key issue is again the building of *some* relationship with the interviewee, and the particular elements of this in dealing with the reluctant client are:

Accept the client's fears.

Accept the client's reluctance as another piece of behaviour to be examined.

Accept the client's reluctance as a consequence of their past interactions, and therefore as normal.

Look for an initial area where agreement can occur and negotiate around this area.

Search for the particular motivations and strengths which apply to this client.

Reinforce compliance in the areas which *can* be negotiated.

AGGRESSION IN INTERVIEWS

When clients become aggressive, this represents a particular challenge to all interviewers, in part because of the strong emotions they generate within us. As a result, dealing effectively with aggression in an interview is an extremely complicated exercise, and one about which many chapters have been written and many workshops held. The reader who is particularly interested in working with such clients is advised to examine Jeremy Coid's chapter in Roslyn Corney's book (Coid, 1991), as a readable introduction, and Farrell & Gray's excellent, sympathetic book (1992) on the topic, which offers a great deal in the way of important skills for managing aggression. For the present, I aim once again simply to offer a list of very basic survival tactics, in recognition of the fact that aggression, like any emotion, can occur in any interview, and, therefore, requires handling by the interviewer. Aggression in interviews is, however, mercifully rare.

Minimize the likelihood that aggression will occur by adherence to the guidelines concerning respect for client's and keeping the client orientated during the interview.

Be aware of the effect of aggressive behaviour on our own emotions, and avoid compounding the problem by displaying aggressive behaviour in return.

Adopt submissive postures in response to aggressive episodes.

Gently share with the client the effect that the aggressive behaviour has upon you.

Invite discussion of the source of the client's hostility, primarily using open questions.

Avoid taking sides or offering detailed justifications of one's position. These are mistaken because they respond on a factual level to emotional issues. The time for explanation is once the aggression has been defused.

Reinforce periods of non-aggression with attentive non-verbal and verbal behaviour.

If an aggressive outburst is thought likely before the interview (for example on the basis of a client's history), plan appropriately by adopting a series of contingency plans for the interview and arranging seating for escape and the availability of others for support.

Avoid over-reacting to histories of aggression, by adopting overly-defensive plans.

If aggression continues or escalates to a level where you feel insufficiently safe, or insufficiently able to concentrate on the process and conduct of the interview, terminate the interview speedily.

CONCLUSION

This concludes our examination of cognitive-behavioural approaches to assessment interviewing. It has been stressed throughout that the approach itself represents but one way of thinking about client difficulties, albeit an extremely well-tested one. In the exercises that follow, therefore, it is extremely important that you adapt and change the details of assessment to fit the approach to patient difficulties with which you are most familiar. Of course, if the cognitive-behavioural elements described in our discussion of conditioning theory, or the associated approaches to treatment are themselves of interest, by all means experiment with these, too. Above all, it is the logical *structure* of the cognitive behavioural assessment that is likely to be useful in the greatest range of situations. I have stressed the importance of client ownership of treatment. The same is true of your ownership of the assessment process, and it is only by constant adaptation of and reflection upon the strategies presented here that such ownership can be gained. The exercises are meant as a starting point for such ownership.

EXERCISES

1 Consider *three* therapeutic interventions in which you are currently involved. Using the section on rationale-giving, write brief notes on how you will transmit a sufficiently detailed rationale to the client to orientate her to the type of treatment being offered and to allow for the giving of informed consent.

2 Review the information on goal-setting, and consider some possible goals for use with clients in your area of clinical expertise, stating them according to the guidelines in Figure 5.3

3 Devise scales to enable the client to measure progress towards these targets.

4 Review the aims and objectives of assessment interviewing described in Chapter 4, and examine your reflective notes from Exercise 3 for that chapter. Specify which *two* of the aims are most important for you to examine at this stage in your evolving interviewing skill. (Remember that to attempt to work on every aspect of interviewing at once will very likely lead to an overload of information, and, in consequence, to unjustified pessimism about the likelihood of success.) Formulate a target statement for each of the aims, using the guidelines for effective baseline measurement given in Figure 5.3, and devise some scale by

which to measure them. Set a timescale for improvement. Do baseline measurements for each target.

5 Allowing plenty of time for the unfamiliarity of the situation, perform an assessment interview with a client, adhering to the guidelines on assessment interviewing offered in this and the previous chapter *to a sufficient degree to allow you to address the targets you have specified in Exercise 4*. Thus, if your targets all relate to information-gathering using the cognitive-behavioural framework, you can proceed according to your normal practice after this stage in the interview has been passed. Similarly, if many of your goals relate to process skills, you may find it best to avoid changing to a consideration of cognitive-behavioural *components* until a later interview, so as to avoid being distracted from the process-oriented targets. If your targets relate to rationale-giving, you will need to ensure that you are adequately prepared (for example, by working through Exercise 1), and so on.

6 Measure your targets again, and reflect upon the process of the interview you performed.

7 Draw up an action plan related to improving assessment interviewing skills. Generate and measure a target for each component of the action plan.

8 Devise action plans for increasing the effectiveness of your communication with:

   a reluctant client;
   an aggressive client.

9 Read Ellis's paper regarding irrational beliefs of therapists. What irrational statements of your own would you add? Are there *positive* as well as negative aspects to having such beliefs? Beware of the addition I made to Ellis's list on page 83)! *Note*: Ellis's paper may be difficult to get if you do not have access to a good nursing, medical or other academic library. If so, Dryden & Ellis (1986) contains an accurate summary of Ellis's paper.

FURTHER READING

Egan, G. (1990) *The Skilled Helper: A Systematic Approach to Effective Helping*. Pacific Grove, California. Brooks/Cole.

Ellis, A. (1983) How to deal with your most difficult client: You. *Journal of Rational-Emotive Therapy* 1 (1), 3-8.

Hawton, K. Salkovskis, P.M. Kirk, J. & Clark, D.M. (eds) *Cognitive-Behaviour Therapy for Psychiatric Problems. A Practical Guide*. Oxford. Oxford University Press.

6   Educating and advising

So far in this book, we have examined how the interviewer can employ effective strategies to maximize the possibility of gaining appropriate information from the client, in order to help in coming to an understanding of her problem. Most interview situations are, of course, a two-way flow of information, and we have touched on this by our discussion of the interviewer's role in facilitating the client's discourse. In this sense, we have already begun to examine some of the important factors involved in advising and educating clients, since much effective eliciting of information follows similar rules to its transmission. In nursing, as in many expert activities, the issues of advice-giving and education often shade into a single pursuit (Bille, 1981). Although the expression 'education' is, in large part, taken to mean the offering of factual information, it is clear that elements of advising come into this activity, as soon as the nurse begins to make the information *personal* to the particular client with whom she is dealing. Since much effective education involves this personalizing of the message, many education textbooks (Quinn, 1988) incorporate discussions of advising and even counselling as part of the educational role. This chapter recognizes the complementary nature of the informative, advice-giving, exploratory and supportive roles, but concentrates primarily on elements which concern information transmission and enhancing the likelihood of the client's understanding and, if so desired, acting on that information. For this reason, I shall, whilst recognizing this complementary nature, refer to such pursuits as informative interviews.

Since a good deal of the information in this chapter relates to the organization of communication with the client, many of the comments in Chapter 5 about the process of the assessment interview are highly relevant. In particular, you may now care to review or re-read the discussions of orientating the client, of goal-setting and the use of reinforcement, particularly as it relates to client coping. In Chapter 4, we discussed the use of aims and objectives during interviewing. As a review, let us use this format again, by setting aims and objectives for the informative interview and using these to organize the chapter. In Chapters 7 and 8, the formulation of aims and objectives will be *your* job, as part of the exercises.

Aims

1 To offer the client understandable information.
2 To offer the client retainable information.
3 To offer the client information in a way which maximizes her personal choice.
4 To offer information collaboratively.
5 To maximize the likelihood that the information offered will be acceptable to the client.

Objectives

1 To identify and address blocks to the learning process.
2 To organize information within an informative interview to take account of memory and motivation aspects of learning.
3 To use visual aids appropriately.
4 To use a personal knowledge base appropriately.
5 To admit areas of ignorance openly and decide on relevant activity.
6 To negotiate agendas of interim learning goals with clients.
7 To assist the client in carrying out agreed instructions.

In Chapter 3, we touched briefly on the work of Donald Schon (1983) with regard to reflection about practice. In developing his model of reflective practice, Schon describes two 'worlds' of client consultation – Model 1 and Model 2. Model 1 behaviour by consultants is characterized by an adversarial stance, which seeks to maintain professional elitism and 'expertise', whilst Model 2 behaviour is essentially collaborative, aiming to maximize choice. Cognitive-behavioural approaches to the informative interview are negotiative in this way, although the interviewer accepts that she may, at times, have specialist information about what is happening to the client, but of which the client is currently unaware. Skilled interviewing introduces this issue into the negotiative process, sometimes through didactic teaching, at others through the process of Socratic questioning described later in this chapter. The aims and objectives offered here are intended to reflect a predominantly Model 2 view of the informative interview. Thus, although we shall be discussing the notion of 'compliance' with therapeutic instructions, advice and educational strategies, compliance refers throughout to the client's carrying out tactics which have been negotiated with the interviewer in accordance with the Model 2 aims of maximizing choice, ownership and involvement. It is accepted that the client's beliefs, attitudes and life circumstances may make compliance difficult, even though the client *wishes* to go along with our advice in the informative interview, and that, in this sense, compliance generation is an enabling and empowering intervention.

Behaviourists have a number of theories of learning based on conditioning principles. We examined these principles in Chapter 4, during our discussion of their role in mediating information-gathering during assessment. Behaviourists see no distinction between formal and informal learning settings, and indeed, regard learning as something which occurs all the time, and is demonstrated by changes in behaviour in response to the forces of operant and classical conditioning. Operant conditioning (the systematic application of rewards and punishments) is seen as being particularly important, because of its ability to elicit new behaviours through the process of shaping (the offer of rewards for each successive approximation to a desired behaviour). In formal teaching situations, therefore, it is important to offer plentiful social reward for the demonstration of new learning. According to behavioural theory, this reinforcement gives rise not only to increased recall of the information learnt, but also to an increase in the activity of *learning*. Here, a nurse checks her client's understanding of medication instructions, using questioning:

Nurse: So just tell me, so that I know I've explained it properly, about your medication?

Client: I have to take two tablets three times a day, but it's important that I take it with food, because otherwise it can lead to stomach upsets.

Nurse: Excellent, well done. That's absolutely right.

This is a very simple example. However, we often require clients to learn quite complex information, whether that be a physiotherapy or exercise routine, a relaxation programme, exposure therapy for phobias, complex self-medication procedures or the care of prostheses. In all these cases, the client may well, in the early stages, need guidance through each stage of the procedure, shaping performance by differential social reward of each correct piece of performance. Incorrect performances are not rewarded, and may be either corrected or ignored by the nurse. Ignoring may be used where formal correction is judged to be too demoralizing, and where further incorrect performances can be allowed to die a natural death in the absence of reinforcement. Where further incorrect performance would be dangerous, prompt correction is clearly needed. In the example below, the nurse has offered and demonstrated to the client a series of breathing exercises as a relaxation tactic. As the client practises the exercises, the nurse refrains from commenting on inappropriate performance, but waits until the occurrence of small positive aspects of performance, and reinforces these heavily, whilst providing information on precisely *what* is being reinforced.

Client: (Breathing quickly, then slows down.)

Nurse: Good, that's slower.

Client: (Continues breathing slowly.)

Nurse: Good.

Client: (Starts to breath too deeply.)

Nurse: (Silence.)

Client: (Breathes more gently.)

Nurse: Good. Gently does it.

In this way it is possible for the nurse to 'shape up' perfect performance of the breathing exercises, without ever punishing inappropriate performance, through social reinforcement. Individuals differ in their ability to tolerate criticism, and cognitive theorists emphasize the importance of feedback rather than reinforcement. Most interviewers will use a mixture of both, but ineffective interviewers offer a great deal of negative feedback, without reinforcement and without offering strategies to help in effective change.

It can be seen, then, that the principles of behavioural approaches to formal teaching and learning are precisely the same as behaviourist approaches to other elements of our experience of and adaptation to the environment. Furthermore, each element of teaching through maximization of the precepts of behavioural learning through reinforcement is similar to the rewarding of client attempts at coping we discussed in Chapter 4. More cognitively-oriented approaches go beyond this, however, and we shall examine these now.

COGNITIVE APPROACHES TO LEARNING AND TEACHING

So far in this book, we have, whilst espousing a cognitive-behavioural account of human experiences, pursued primarily a *behavioural* approach to the *techniques* of human interaction, emphasizing the most effective ways of organizing the interview so as to offer appropriate reinforcement to the client. Examination of cognitive elements has been confined to our general approach to the client and to the content of our assessment, goal-setting and intervention. In the informative interview, however, there are a number of insights from information-processing theories which can help with effective client education.

I have argued elsewhere (Newell & Dryden, 1991) that cognitive theories arose in part in responses to weaknesses in behaviourism, particularly its difficulty in accounting for complex learning phenomena, such as language (Chomsky, 1959). Probably the first therapist to break from strict behavioural theories was Albert Bandura (1977a), whose *social learning theory* we encountered briefly in Chapter 1. You will remember that Bandura's distinctive contribution was to demonstrate that humans and animals learnt not only through the processes of the offering of rewards and punishments, but also through observation of the application of those rewards and punishments to others. In the same way that we are more likely to perform again an activity that has been rewarded by others or the environment, so we are more likely to perform an activity for which we have seen another person being rewarded. Thus, in education, this *vicarious learning* is a potent source of motivation for learners. In the informative interview, we have the opportunity to offer clients examples of the likely consequences of remembering and using information we have offered, and can also offer them the example of other successful clients. The more closely we can make the example fit the client's own situation, the more likely that they will benefit from the effects of this modelling. Although interviewers themselves can be powerful models for clients, their effectiveness is lessened by the simple fact that they *are* professionals, and therefore are perceived by clients as coping. In order to be truly effective models, interviewers need to take careful account of the client's personal circumstances, and use self-disclosure (see Chapter 7) to close the gap between themselves as models and the client. If the client needs help in remembering information, the offer of examples of how other clients, and the interviewer herself, have used particular tactics, and the beneficial consequences, may be useful (symbolic modelling). If the learning required is more concerned with motor skills or experiences, as in our example of learning a breathing exercise, demonstration and simulation may be required, but again with the addition of examples of successful clients. In the best of situations, the interviewer encourages the client to act as her *own model*, by remembering examples from her own life of skills she has used which are similar to those required currently, whether these be motor skills, coping tactics or tricks of memorization. In this kind of *'automodelling'*, the client should also recall the positive consequences of the tactics she employed. Finally, symbolic models, which offer some written or other inanimate representation of the required performance can also be offered, again with reference to reinforcing consequences.

Clearly, in learning, motivation is of considerable importance, and we may describe compliance with therapeutic instructions as a function of memory of the information received and the motivation to carry out the instructions contained in that information. Modelling is one way of both increasing the likelihood that instructions will be retained *and* carried out, and much of the information in this chapter relates to the enhancement of client motivation in these two ways, as did our discussion of the application of direct reinforcement. I think it is fair, however, to regard conditioning and social learning processes as being *primarily* concerned with motivation, whereas the cognitive theories we will deal with in the following paragraphs are concerned mainly with how information is organized by teacher and learner, and the impact of this organization on retention and recall.

In discussing social learning, we noted the importance of internal representations of the world in client learning. According to social learning theory, the individual builds up a series of pictures of the likely future consequences of her actions, and acts according to whether or not reinforcement is likely to be forthcoming. Cognitive theories emphasise even more strongly the importance of these internal representations, and describe the individual as primarily a processor of information. In this processing, there is a dynamic relationship between memory, perception and cognition. The mind is organized in a categorical way, according to sets of rules which mediate the relationships between categories and the objects in each category (Collins & Quillian, 1972). As a result, effective teaching needs to take account of the way such categories are organized, and effective learning involves the acquisition of new concepts and categories, as well as new 'facts'.

In Chapter 3, we discussed the role of memory in reflection, and much of this information is again relevant in the context of the informative interview. Thus, the effective interviewer offers copious links between the acquisition phase (the informative interview) and the retrieval phase (the context in which performance is required). In this way, the effects of state- and context-dependency, and of the interpolation of other unrelated material, are reduced. Written material can be of great value here (Ley, 1984). This may be especially useful if the client is herself responsible for the preparation of such material, through note-taking, or the completion of self-completion handouts which provide headings to assist client recall. Once again, there is a motivational aspect here, since the client is herself responsible for her learning, a factor recognized as increasing retention and compliance. With regard to transfer of training to the client's life away from the interview, the use of written material, however brief, has the additional advantage of changing the job of remembering instructions from one of recall to the easier task of recognition. Once again, we see the similarity between clients and ourselves, since, as with professional reflection, the use of checklists of all kinds can perform a similar function in aiding the client's memory and orienting her to the appropriate tactics to be used in performance situations away from the interview.

Further practical aids are the use of mnemonics, schemes which enable the client to think of the information to be remembered by the use of some kind of cognitive linking device. Many of these are familiar to us all. Richard Of York Gave Battle In Vain is known to all children as a means of remembering the sequence of the colours of the rainbow. Since meaningful information is better recalled than meaningless (Jung, 1968), this kind of natural language mediation of recall works by imparting meaning to an otherwise meaningless string of words (Red, Orange, Yellow, etc.). The use of rhymes works according to the same principle. Similarly, acronyms (words in which each letter is the first letter of a word to be remembered) are such a widely-recognized means of remembering information that organizations are often at great pains to invent titles which translate well into acronymic form. Indeed, the ABCs model of assessment is itself an acronym. Although ABC is not, strictly speaking, a word, it is wordlike in structure, since we talk of 'learning our ABCs'. It has the additional advantage that the acronym itself reflects something about its content (fundamentals). Arnold Lazarus (1973), a prominent eclectic behaviourist, has BASIC ID as the acronym for his assessment strategy in multimodal therapy, again reflecting the content of the words – discovering the basic identity of the client and her problems. This again adds meaning to the information, and also *organizes* and *simplifies* it. A further commonly-used technique is the method of loci, where each item to be remembered is mentally located at some particular point in a place well-known to the client. To recall the information, the client 'walks through' the place in her mind and retrieves the information. This memory technique has a long history in oral traditions, before the written word became available to large sections of the population. Generally speaking, this technique is most useful in the recall of brief, specific pieces of factual information. Finally, the client can use 'linkword' techniques, linking the information to be remembered with some striking image which can be readily associated with it. For example, medication times might be associated with the hands of the clock, the vividness being increased by client imagining looking at a favourite family heirloom watch and chain. Once again the use of this technique may be limited to relatively simple information. In all the above techniques, the nature of the associations may be quite bizarre. This is not important, as long as meaning is preserved or enhanced and structure simplified. In fact, the unusual content of the mnemonics may itself enhance memory by increasing the salience of the information in memory, by virtue of its novel quality. It is likely that the greater the role played by clients themselves in constructing mnemonics, the greater the enhancement of recall, since construction of mnemonics implies a further elaboration of meaning, further routes to encoding in memory, repetition of content and greater relevance of the mnemonic to the client.

Over and above these tactics, we can, during the interview, offer the client information in ways which optimize the use of her cognitive structures. This can be done by drawing on empirical studies of the process of remembering information. As part of his numerous investigations of the relationship between clinicians and clients, Philip Ley (1976), whose name has cropped up several times during this book, has conducted many examinations of how information is recalled by clients, and has offered a number of solutions to client difficulties in recalling the information offered by clinicians. He found that four tactics resulted in greater recall of information by clients: the use of shorter words and sentences, repetition, explicit categorization and specific rather than general statements. To the first of these ideas might be added the notion of *linguistic congruence*, in which the interviewer attends to and adopts certain verbal expressions of the client. This may very well involve the use of shorter words and simpler sentence constructions, but could, in the case of a well-educated client, or one with specialist knowledge, involve using quite complex advice couched in terms familiar to the client, for example, using analogies from science with an engineer, from play with a child, from painting with an artist, and so on. In all instances, however, the interviewer tries to match her discourse with the client's cognitive abilities and set as accurately as possible. *Repetition* is a simple tactic, which depends for its effectiveness both on increased chances of the client's having attended appropriately to the information and increased opportunities for transfer of it into memory. This may be particularly important, since the client's attention may be diminished during the interview by the effect of anxiety. As an addition, repetition by the client has the added advantage of being an active process, allowing the client to repeat the information in her own words (increasing relevance) and allowing the interviewer to check understanding. Repetition of this kind, or overlearning, is a well-verified component of behavioural approaches to therapy, and appears to confer some resistance to forgetting upon the overlearnt information. Explicit categorization needs a little explanation, and is, in essence, offering the client a series of contextual cues which enable her to isolate the information presented in a discrete category in memory, by explaining the order in which information will be presented and what the focus of each piece of information will be. In fact, the example of initial orientation of the client to the interview process given in Chapter 2 is an example of explicit categorization. Another is given in the case material at the end of this chapter. The giving of *specific, rather than general, information* involves the offering of concrete examples of what is required of the client, and is very similar to the behavioural goal-setting we have already examined, in that it should possess precise descriptions of what is required of the client or of what will happen to the client. Thus, it is inappropriate to advise: ' You must cut down on your drinking' from an information transfer viewpoint, as well as because of the dogmatic nature of the advice. After appropriate negotiation, the advice: 'You must drink no more than two pints of bitter each night' is much better. As we will see when we discuss interim targets later in this chapter, the client now knows exactly what is expected, and can make a reasonable decision about whether or not to participate, but, additionally, the information is simply more likely to be recalled.

In addition to the four aspects of information presentation identified by Ley, a number of general rules about presentation can enhance client recall. Attention to the order in which information is presented will pay dividends in terms of client recall. Information presented at the end of a period of information acquisition (e.g. a teaching session, a list of articles to be recalled) is recalled best (Gregg, 1986). Thus items presented at the end of a list of items are better recalled than those presented at the beginning or in the middle of the list, though the effect is quickly lost. Items presented at the beginning of the list are also recalled well, and this effect is more durable. Items presented in the middle are recalled least well. Thus, skilled interviewers present important information near the beginning of an interview and reprise it at the end. Proceeding from the *general to the specific*, which we mentioned in talking about information-gathering, is useful in information transmission, too, since clients are provided with general structures into which to place the specific information offered. This is similar to Ausubel's ideas about the use of advance organizers in teaching (Ausubel *et al.*, 1978), and also represents a more general example of Ley's notion of explicit categorization, since it is another way in which the interviewer provides categories in order to assist recall. If we can enhance this categorization by the use of striking stimuli (e.g. visual aids), the usefulness of this categorization in recall is also likely to be increased.

We mentioned repetition and overlearning as a means making information more resistant to forgetting. Practice of behaviours to be performed provides much the same function, especially where motor skills are involved. We encountered this use of *rehearsal* in our examination of reflection. For clients, as for interviewers, rehearsal provides plentiful opportunities for reinforcement, both from others and from ourselves, rendering it more likely that the rehearsed behaviour will occur in situations away from the interview. In addition, anyone who has attempted to learn to play a musical instrument will attest to the value of rehearsal in helping us to remember crucial information at some later time, particularly when under stress. A final element of practice is the incorporation of *theoretical* material into some practical setting, as soon as possible after it has been acquired. The practical application of theory in this way aids its retention in memory, which illustrates the reasoning behind our progression from general to specific examples in rationale-giving during cognitive-behavioural assessment. Demonstrations of the practical usefulness of theoretical information not only help provide links with existing knowledge (itself an important factor in maximizing memory), but also offer reinforcement for remembering, since the client can see the likely consequences of the theory in practice. One special kind of rehearsal involves the use of *Socratic questioning* in teaching, in which the interviewer asks the client a series of questions which are designed to lead the client into a position of demonstrating to herself the logic of certain ideas about her difficulties or ways of proceeding in addressing these problems. For example, the interviewer may ask the client to relate how a general rationale applies to some specific situation which she finds problematic, continually asking what the client should do next, and why. As a result the client (a) is more likely to put the ideas into practice, (b) has the opportunity for additional verbal rehearsal of the appropriate ideas and (c) receives the reinforcement of having arrived at the ideas herself. A major variant of cognitive therapy relies heavily on Socratic questioning (Beck, 1976).

OTHER ASPECTS OF COMPLIANCE

We have noted that compliance is affected both by memory and by motivation, and have dealt so far with interventions which affect both, or which work by enhancing memory alone. To finish this section, we will now explore some tactics which primarily affect motivation. Most of these return to social learning theory, and offer techniques to increase the client's opportunities for observing appropriate direct and symbolic models.

It should first be noted that rehearsal, which we discussed earlier, is itself a form of automodelling, in which the client performs some approximation to the real-world behaviour which has been agreed, and receives reinforcement for so doing. In social learning terms, the client forms a representation of likely reinforcement for performing the real act. This rehearsal need not be behavioural, and, indeed, rehearsals of actual behaviour are often impractical, since the actual stimuli which the behaviour addresses are not necessarily available during the interview, and can only rarely be induced artificially. For example, the client learning coping tactics for use with chronic episodic pain can rarely guarantee the occurrence of pain in the clinic. Although I had a certain amount of success in training clients to artificially induce pain, using the imagination (Newell, 1987), and much hypnotherapy uses such techniques, very often some rehearsal which does not involve the actual stimulus is required. In this case, 'talk-throughs', 'walk-throughs', 'think-throughs' and even 'write throughs' can all act as symbolic models for the client, with appropriate reinforcement being offered by the interviewer. Talk-throughs and think-throughs are straightforward enough, requiring the client to imagine each aspect of a problematic situation, whilst walk-throughs are essentially mimes of required behaviours in the absence of the actual stimulus. Write-throughs can involve practice of the completion of diaries and other forms of recording, or written notes on the client's performance which she takes away from the interview into the situation where performance is required.

As a variant on these techniques, the client can be encouraged to *self-reinforce*, either by stating how well they have done and why, or by imagining the positive consequences of compliance, in terms of decreased handicap, the good opinion of others, and so on. This self-reinforcement is a powerful way of generating compliance, and should be encouraged wherever possible, both during rehearsal and in the actual situation. The role of the interviewer here is to help the client to identify appropriate reinforcers. A further method is encouraging the client to identify all the difficulties associated with non-compliance. Clients are often well aware of such difficulties, but neglect their existence because confrontation of our difficulties appears much more threatening in the short-term. Identifying long-term consequences of not confronting helps the client to create a mental or written '*balance-sheet*', which aids in decision-making about whether change is more desirable than staying the same. As a final approach, the interviewer can introduce the idea of *contracting*, in which the client agrees to perform certain behaviours, in return for certain behaviours by the interviewer, or in return for certain agreed changes in the environment (e.g. that pain will decrease to within certain limits after so long an attempt at practising pain control strategies). This contract can be either informal and verbal or formal and written.

The above issues are now summarized in Figure 6.1

Use of reinforcement and differential reinforcement to encourage correct recall. Encouragement of self-reinforcement by the client. Use of rehearsal.

Use of actual and symbolic modelling and encouragement of 'automodelling' by the client. Use of written material and other visual aids.

Mnemonics, talk-throughs, walk-throughs, think-throughs and write-throughs.

Short words, repetition, explicit categorization and specific statements.

Proceeding from the general to the specific.

Rehearsal, Socratic questioning, self-reinforcement

Figure 6.1 Maximizing information transmission and compliance during the informative interview

A NOTE ON NON-COMPLIANCE

A the very beginning of this book, we noted the magnitude of the problem of non-compliance with therapeutic instructions, yet there is no specific information here about dealing with non-compliance. This is for two reasons. First, prevention is better than cure, and the bulk of this book is, in fact, concerned with increasing compliance through the use of appropriate interviewing skills.

Through these, we aim to increase the accuracy of the information we receive from clients and increase their role in negotiating intervention, their understanding of what is required of them and their satisfaction with the interview. Second, in cognitive-behavioural terms, non-compliance as a problem is no different from any other difficulty clients present with. As a result, the best way of approaching non-compliance is by assessing it using the ABC model, exactly as if it were any other piece of client behaviour.

INTERIM GOALS

During our examination of compliance, we spoke of contracting with clients. In some senses, every part of the informative interview requires informal contracting, since there is either implicit or explicit negotiation of what the client will do to address her difficulties. As before, the line between education and advising is very slim, but in almost all informative interviews some behaviour change will be required of the client. A key element in the generation of compliance is that this behaviour change should be negotiated with the client. This involves the setting with the client of interim goals or objectives. These goals are formed in exactly the same way as the intervention outcome goals we described in Chapter 5, and thus possess the same qualities of desirability to the client, practicality, representativeness of other changes and expressivity of significant change in themselves. Furthermore, goals should also be stated in the behavioural terms stated in Figure 5.3. As a result of this emphasis on precision, difficulties in deciding when a desired interim goal has been achieved, and, therefore, when to move to the next such goal, should be minimized.

However, one major difference with interim goals is their much more focal nature. Since interim goals are required to be achieved over a much shorter period of time, both the difficulty and breadth of such goals need to be much less than is expressed in outcome goals. Moreover, interim goals will probably not have the same amount of desirability for the client as outcome goals, particularly since interim goals often have low representativeness, relating to the *process* of intervention rather than representing something the client ultimately wants to achieve. It is possible to offer interim goals for some clients which *do* represent real changes (for example the agoraphobic who agrees to walk to Tesco's by the end of the week), but not for others (like the completion of a specified number of exercises by the obese client, in the absence of weight loss). This may be a cause of poor compliance, especially if the achievement of the interim goal requires a good deal of effort. As a result, the construction of interim goals requires sensitivity and perseverance to find the most *potentially* rewarding interim goal for a given client at a given stage in the intervention. This generally represents a small but significant 'next step' for the client in the process of addressing her difficulties.

Several useful 'rules of thumb' can be employed here. First, *always set goals which relate to outcome*. Given what we have said in the previous paragraph, this seems like a logical impossibility, but one can, for example, set several related interim goals, some of which relate to process, whilst others represent concrete steps towards treatment outcome goals. Thus, for the obese client above, her goals of exercising a certain number of times can be paired with a goal of losing a certain amount of weight as a result of calorific restriction. Second, *link process goals to outcome*. This can be done through verbal explanation:

Nurse: The point about doing these exercises is that, even though we can't expect it to result in much weight loss at this stage, it does relate to the overall lack of fitness which we identified as part of your difficulties.

An alternative is to allow the client to make this link, with encouragement and guidance from the interviewer, perhaps using the Socratic questioning mentioned earlier.

Third, *emphasize the rewarding consequences of adhering to process goals*, using the rehearsal and automodelling tactics we described earlier. Fourth, *allow the client to lead the process* of deciding upon the next step to be attempted. Fifth, *guide the client towards the optimally reinforcing goal* available at a given time. This is an issue of helping the client to decide how much they can achieve at a given time, so that they do not miss the opportunity for the most powerful reinforcement from themselves and others, but do not attempt a task which they have little likelihood of achieving. The interviewer offers the client a process of risk assessment, combined with a profit/loss examination. Sixth, *set a variety of goals of different difficulty*. In this way, the client is always assured of some degree of success. This is part of a process of contingency planning. Clearly, interviewers and clients alike are reluctant to predict failure in the performance of the contracted activities. However, the inclusion of the client in the therapeutic endeavour involves the admission of the possibility that things will sometimes go better, at other times worse, during treatment. As a result, each goal should have a series of success criteria, which allow for 'fall-back' positions when things do not go well. Once again, the client is assured of some degree of success in all but the most disastrous of scenarios. The client herself may be able to offer valuable advice about the best such fall-back arrangements. In this setting, the talk-through procedures we discussed earlier have an additional advantage in helping to alert client and interviewer to possible difficulties in the performance of instructions away from the clinic, and possible coping strategies can then be discussed. A final consideration about interim goals is that, unlike treatment outcome goals, they often involve the *interviewer*, as well as the client, in some kind of behaviour away from the interview setting. Whether this is a minimal intervention, such as being available for telephone advice at given times, or represents a significant input on the part of the interviewer, such as negotiating the availability of special equipment or resources, this should be explicitly negotiated and contracted with the client. Thus, as a seventh suggestion: *state proposed interviewer behaviour precisely*. As a result, client trust in the interviewer is likely to be increased. This itself may have a beneficial effect on compliance.

The combination of the above elements represents a way of involving the client at each stage of the process of interim goal-setting, and maximizes her control of the intervention process, allowing the specification of next steps and contingency planning to remain substantially in her hands. Nevertheless, the interviewer also has rights in this process, since, as we have noted, negotiation is a reciprocal arrangement. Thus, if the interviewer believes, after having followed all the suggestions above, that the interim goals selected by the client are either so unreasonable as to be incapable of being met, or so modest in terms of the change they represent that they are unlikely to have any impact on the client's difficulties, then confrontation of this behaviour, with the aim of re-negotiating interim goals, is required (see Figure 6.2).

Set goals that relate to outcome.

Link process goals to outcome.

Emphasize the rewards of process goals.

Allow the client to lead the process.

Guide the client to the optimally rewarding goal.

Set a variety of goals of differing difficulty.

State interviewer behaviour explicitly.

Figure 6.2 Setting interim goals

RESOURCES FOR THE INFORMATIVE INTERVIEW

The first such resource is the interviewer herself: her experiences, attitudes and, above all, knowledge of the information to be imparted. The experiences and attitudes of the interviewer are of great importance in facilitating the transmission of information, and personal experiences can, in addition, form part of the body of knowledge which the interviewer offers the client, in the form of real life examples of the general principles she offers the client. Nevertheless, these important elements of teaching are of little value without a sound grasp of the subject matter of the informative interview. Therefore, informative interviews which are successful are carried out by people who have access to suitable resources to become expert in their subject. These include institutional libraries, meetings with professional colleagues both locally and at national and inter-national conferences, and *time*. All these things are difficult to negotiate within institutional contexts, where the institution may have priorities which are very different from those of the clinician and the client. One method here is to begin in a small way – the foot in the door technique – by applying to the interviewer's superiors for a relatively insignificant outlay on either material resources or support for personal development, and attempting to demonstrate the effect that such an outlay will have on efficacy in interactions with clients, or in cascading of training to other staff. Larger requests can then be based on the employer's reaction to these earlier reports. Most managers are prepared to support staff to some degree if they see they are getting something tangible in return for their support. Nevertheless, it is acknowledged that seeking funding for courses to enrich one's clinical expertise is an arduous process. However, of all the resources sought, time is the most precious. In case management terms, time spent in preparation is never wasted, and this is particularly true in the case of the informative interview. In formal education, it takes many hours to develop a single hour of lecture material. Although the informative interview is, generally, a more informal setting in which the area to be covered is smaller and often extremely familiar to the interviewer, 'off-the-cuff' attempts at client teaching are rarely successful, since they fail to take account of individual variables. Thus, the interviewer needs, as a minimum, time to consider how her messages will be put over to the client in the way which is most easily understood and has the most impact for that individual.

Having stated that the interviewer should be an 'expert', it is clear that occasions will arise where the client's questions or even expertise outstrip the knowledge of the interviewer. That this should be an issue of some concern and embarrassment for interviewers is, perhaps, inevitable. However, skilful interviewers who are adopting the Model 2 approach mentioned at the beginning of this chapter use such occurrences as an opportunity to maximize learning for both client and interviewer. In the case of the expert client, the interviewer needs to be willing to learn from the client and incorporate the client's views into the process of the informative interview. That the client is more knowledgeable in certain areas can be used as a source of great reinforcement for the client, and thus as a generator of compliance, providing that the interviewer is frank and willing to learn. A decrease in client confidence is only inevitable if the interviewer retreats into adversarial interviewing techniques in an attempt to preserve professional pride. By contrast, the client whose questions we cannot answer rarely needs more than a frank recognition of this fact, followed with a contract on the part of the interviewer to find out the relevant information. Indeed, client and interviewer can agree that *both* will attempt to find out as much as possible about the problematic question, and compare notes at the next session, thus emphasizing the negotiated, collaborative nature of intervention. Clients rarely expect us to be all-knowing. It is clinicians who expect that of *themselves*, in response to the automatic negative thinking identified by Ellis (1983). Thus, they attempt to protect themselves from threats to this expectation, when this is actually unnecessary.

Both comprehensibility and impact can be enhanced by the use of various teaching aids. Whilst it is beyond the scope of this book to examine this complex subject in any detail, the informative interview is a good setting in which to begin to come to grips with visual aids. As we have noted, the setting is generally informal, and so anxiety on the part of the interviewer is likely to be less than in a large, formal lecture. Also, the kinds of aid suitable for such informal settings are likely to be simple, and thus take less expertise to manipulate effectively. In order to use visual aids appropriately, the interviewer may begin by considering the following issues:

Are the aids adequately prepared? A rushed preparation is unlikely to allow sufficient time for checking the appropriateness of the aids for a particular client.

Are the aids of adequate quality? The whole point of using visual aids is to create an impact on the client which reinforces the interviewer's messages. Poor quality visual aids are unlikely to create the professional impression the interviewer desires in order to increase client confidence.

Do the aids support the points I want to make? If they do not, they are mere distraction, however well they are presented. Similarly, the use of too many aids is distracting rather than focussing.

Am I familiar with the content of the aid? Since clients will be expected to discuss and ask questions about the content of visual aids, familiarity with it is expected of the interviewer.

Is the information contained in the aid correct? Although this seems obvious, many leaflets published by both statutory and voluntary bodies are either incorrect or out-of-date.

Is the information suitable for the client? Suitability may refer to the level of the information contained, which may be either too simple or too complex for a particular client, and to the content of the information, which may contain inappropriate or irrelevant elements. Clients should be alerted to this latter element if an alternative source cannot be selected.

Used with a sensitive consideration of the above points, visual aids can assist the interviewer in transmitting her messages to the client, and interviewers will find it useful to have a personal and constantly reviewed and updated library of leaflets and posters from a variety of organizations, as well as adaptations from such written material to personalize it to an individual client's needs, and graphs and charts to demonstrate clients' continuing progress in achieving their intervention goals. More complex visual aids are also occasionally useful, for example in the use of video recording equipment to show educational films or offer immediate feedback on client performance, or the use of computer-assisted learning packages. In some cases, such as a recent experiment at the Maudsley Hospital Behaviour Therapy Unit in London, computers can be used as an almost complete replacement for the interviewer in assessment and informative interviewing. Although a certain amount of training is necessary to use complex aids of this kind, the general rules stated above regarding their use apply equally. Aids are adapted to fit each client; clients are not adapted to fit aids, however elegant.

This concludes our examination of the informative interview. In the following case material, Angie, a practice nurse, has been working for a few sessions with

Sara, who had a mastectomy a year ago. Sara has avoided a number of activities because of her thoughts about her body. She and Angie have now agreed that Sara will start to resume these activities and have set some treatment outcome goals. We join this interview as Angie is about to review information she has given Sara about the process of anxiety reduction over time, and its effect in helping her to come to terms with altered body image (Newell, 1991), before going on to arrange some interim goals related to Sara's attempts to tackle her difficulties. For the purpose of this example, only those elements of the interview which relate to information transmission and compliance generation have been retained.

CLINICAL EXAMPLE

Angie: Let me just say again (*Repetition.*), then, that the general idea here is that by repeating these avoided activities, you get used to the anxiety they cause. This does mean that you have to do the things which cause anxiety, and do them often. This can be taken a step at a time, though. (*Proceeding from the general to the specific, using short words and sentences.*) Can you tell me what you understand about how we're going to be working together?

Sara: Well, you explained to me how my fears about the way my body looks are maintained because I don't do anything that helps me feel good about my body. For instance, I avoid exercise, swimming, going out socially.

Angie: (Nods) That's right. (*Reinforcement.*) What else?

Sara: That, by confronting the fear, your body gets used to the physical feelings of fear, and you learn through experience that the feeling goes away. You also prove to yourself, by doing, that you can cope with the things you used to be able to do.

Angie: Absolutely spot on. Let's go on now to look at your first treatment goal and how we can work towards it this week and what tactics you're going to use to make sure things go as well as possible. (*Explicit categorisation and use of specifics.*) Just remind me what your first target was. (*Encouraging repetition and verbal rehearsal.*)

Sara: I want to be able to go out with friends, including people who don't know about the mastectomy, and wear fashionable clothes.

Angie: Well remembered. (*Differential reinforcement.*) I think this is an important goal, and I know it gives you a lot of anxiety even to think about it. You remember we spoke about a client I had with similar difficulties? Well, I phoned her, and she said it was OK to discuss her experiences with you. I think it's fair to say she was more scared than you are at the start of treatment, but, by working step by step, she became able to do all the things, socially, that she was able to do before she had her mastectomy. This took a lot of time and courage, but in the end she was successful. From the way we have talked over the last few weeks, you seem to me to be, if anything, even more determined than she was to overcome these difficulties. (*Offering opportunity for vicarious learning.*) Of course, we agreed that it wasn't realistic to ask you to do this all at once. What do you think you would be able to do this week?

Sara: It's difficult. I thought I might be able to go to a pub with John.

Angie: Excellent. That's something you've not done yet. (*Differential reinforcement.*) How many times could you do that?

Sara: Twice?

Angie: Twice is OK, but . . . you remember we talked about the need for frequency in performing these activities, so you could get used to them more quickly? (*Guiding client towards most potentially reinforcing task.*)

Sara: Yes, well, three times?

Angie: Could you manage that?

Sara: (Nods).

Angie: Excellent. One thing I must ask, though, is that you drink something non-alcoholic. Otherwise alcohol will bring your anxiety down, instead of you doing it. I realize it makes it a bit artificial, since your real goal would involve some alcohol, but it is important in order to help develop the skills in coping with anxiety. And you need those skills to reach the eventual goal. (*Linking process goal to outcome.*) Maybe there is some reward you could give yourself for achieving this target, though? (*Encouraging self-reinforcement.*)

Sara: I could have a drink when we got home?

Angie: (Laughs) Sure, but only . . .

Sara: Only after the anxiety has gone down! (Laughs)

Angie: Brilliant! Can you just talk me through how you're going to go about it, then?

(*This is a kind of Socratic question, in which Sara generates her own advice. It also gives Sara the opportunity to talk through the whole evening, including bathing, getting dressed, looking in the mirror, and so on, as well as what happens actually in the pub. At each stage, Angie can help Sara to identify potential difficulties and generate appropriate coping tactics. Sara writes these down for later use away from the interview.*)

Angie: OK, now just to be on the safe side, supposing you find you absolutely can't get out three times during the week. What's your fallback position?

Sara: I could go out somewhere public with John during the day?

Angie: Excellent. Now just remind me of how you're going to feel after you've completed these trips out? (*Using Socratic questioning to encourage Sara to self-model her own future behaviour by describing the reinforcement she will get.*)

Sara: How do you mean?

Angie: You know, what we talked about before. About you and John.

Sara: Oh. Well, it will be such a great feeling to be out doing something with him. Also, he'll be thrilled, which will make me feel happy, too. And it'll be so good to know I've been able to handle it, even though it makes me nervous.

Angie: Great. Now let's just have a look at the notes you've just made (*Emphasizing, through attention, the importance of written material.*), then we'll recap on how to deal with feeling bad while you're out, then we'll finish. (*Explicit categorization, repeating important aspects at end of interview.*)

EXERCISES

1 Using your knowledge of clients in your current area of clinical expertise, construct the following:

An outline for an informative interview for clients about the interventions you offer.
Five possible visual aids to start or continue your personal visual aid repertoire.

2 Examine the notes of a client you have dealt with in the past, where compliance has been a problem, focussing on how far the suggestions made about client memory and motivation enhancement were followed. Construct a plan of how you would deal with this client if they were referred again, so as to increase their involvement and compliance with care.

3 Conduct your next three informative interviews following the suggestions in this chapter. Review your results using the reflective diary.

FURTHER READING

Bille, D.A. (1981) *Practical Approaches to Patient Teaching*. Boston. Little, Brown & Co.
Wilson-Barnett, J. (1983) *Patient Teaching*. Edinburgh. Churchill Livingstone.
Wilson-Barnett, J. (1991) Providing relevant information for patients and their families. *In* R.Corney (ed.) *Developing Communication and Counselling Skills in Medicine*. London. Routledge.

7 Exploring emotions, supporting and consoling

A great deal of this book so far has concerned what the nurse might *do* in a variety of circumstances, and so there has tended to be an emphasis on specific skills. This chapter is no exception, and aims to offer specific pieces of skilled intervention with clients which, together, comprise that sensitive support which, arguably (Sundeen *et al.*, 1989), lies at the core of skilled nursing. This chapter *is* different, however, in that it covers an area that is often associated, by other authors, with qualities or attributes of the nurse.

In Chapter 1, I examined briefly Carl Rogers' (1957) contention that personal qualities of the therapist (warmth, empathy and genuineness) were necessary and sufficient conditions for successful therapy, and the refutation of this by Lambert *et al.* (1978). Indeed, in recent years, a great deal of counselling has moved a good way from Rogers' position, towards more focal, eclectic, directive interventions. Nevertheless, the emphasis on the personal qualities of the therapist has continued to enjoy considerable currency in the nursing literature. Cognitive-behaviourists believe that all humans possess the positive characteristics identified by Rogers, and as we noted in the introductory material, cognitive-behaviour therapists also demonstrate these characteristics in their attitude to the nurse–client relationship, and their assumptions about the client. There are, however, two important qualifications to this belief in the intrinsic openness, warmth and empathy of humans. The first is that such attributes are only likely to be demonstrated in situations with which the nurse feels relatively comfortable or confident, and the second is that the demonstration of such attributes is a matter of skilled performance, and that, just like any other skill, can be carried out with more or less expertise. To put it another way, it does not matter how caring the nurse is, the client will never benefit from this if the nurse is either too anxious or too socially unskilled to demonstrate her caring nature.

Regarding the first issue, we discussed anxiety to some degree in our examination of reflection and the need to learn through practice. In addition to this, increasing skills in the process of interviewing are also a potent source of anxiety reduction, as confidence grows. However, the area of emotion handling, which is central to the processes of support, requires particular skill in being able to *be* with the client without the luxury of having very much to *do*. In order to do this, a certain amount of willingness to examine one's own anxiety levels and to tolerate some discomfort in the presence of clients are required

Given that one has this willingness, practice of such examination of your interviews will lead to reasonably rapid anxiety reduction. This, however, is only a beginning, since it does not matter how far one feels free to empathise with the client, or how aware one is of the effect of the client's emotions on one's own inner life, if that empathy cannot be transmitted to the client in a way which has meaning for her, and here we return to the idea of skilled performance in the transmission to the client of those elements of one's personality and training which enable us to offer support and consolation, which is what the bulk of this chapter is all about. Thus, by the end of the chapter, you should have a sound grasp of how to go about demonstrating to clients understanding of their difficulties, willingness to participate in their efforts to come to terms with such difficulties and availability to offer support during those efforts and reassurance and commiseration when things are not going well.

So far, we have encountered the idea of the nurse as a very active participant: a leader and a teacher, as well as a partner in client care. We have, therefore, spent a good deal of time looking at how the nurse goes about gathering information and using it to plan with the client the interventions likely to be of use to her. As well as such information processing skills, the ability to *handle emotion* is fundamental to nursing interventions. Here I am using the word 'fundamental' in its precise sense, as being something which is at the bottom or foundation of other aspects of caring. This does not give it priority over, say, choice of appropriate intervention techniques in terms of importance in effecting change in a client. Rather, the ability to handle the flow of emotion between nurse and client is an enabling and enhancing skill. There is no doubt that even in its absence clients will continue to benefit from appropriate advice, as attempts to automate cognitive-behavioural interventions have demonstrated, for example, through the use of computers (Ghosh *et al.*, 1988) and self-help books (Mathews *et al.*, 1977). Nevertheless, such issues of relationship between client and clinician have been repeatedly demonstrated to form an important variable in determining response to interventions. Compliance with therapeutic instructions and client satisfaction are both related to client perceptions of the clinician (Ley, 1977, 1982).

It is also often the case that the nurse can actually *do* very little for the client, either because the answer to the client's difficulties lie so clearly in the client's sight that all the nurse has to do is get out of the light and help the client see it, because the client knows perfectly well what must be done and requires nothing more than permission in order to do it, or because the nature of her difficulties means that nothing can be done. In each of these situations, however, there are a number of things the nurse can *be* which can facilitate the client.

ACTIVE LISTENING SKILLS

Much of what we talked about during Chapter 5 concerned the facilitation of conversation with the client through the use of skills which rewarded information, and many of these issues are common to the supportive elements of interviewing, too. It may be useful, therefore, to revisit some of these elements now, by rereading parts of Chapter 5. In particular, redirecting, summarizing and questioning also form an important part of our repertoire in facilitating the expression of emotion during exploration, support and consolation. For this reason, they are discussed again briefly later in this chapter.

Most nurses have received some instruction in interaction skills, and a number of good texts exist (e.g. Brammer, 1988; Burnard & Morrison, 1991). Although I do not propose to cover that ground again in this book, it may be useful to examine again some major aspects of these skills, in the context of the supportive interview, and viewed primarily from a cognitive-behavioural perspective.

ATTENDING TO NON-VERBAL COMMUNICATION

Here the nurse may ask one simple question: 'What does this person's non-verbal communication tell me about their feelings?' Although some aspects of non-verbal communication are universal (Ekman & Friesen, 1971), there is little doubt that others are highly culture-bound. Interviewers need to bear this in mind in their deliberations, and temper their assumptions accordingly. Even though it is unrealistic to expect busy clinicians to have a working knowledge of the nuances of non-verbal communication from many cultures, it is, equally, the responsibility of interviewers who work extensively with particular ethnic and cultural groups to have knowledge both of differences in characteristic non-verbal behaviours and verbal idioms. Robert Liberman (1975), discussing social skills training, gives a wonderful example of a hand gesture, generally taken to mean 'OK!' which is, to Hispanic Americans, an invitation to perform a sexual act! Unfortunately for the interviewer, not all such confusions are so readily resolved.

Even excluding the issue of cultural norms, which exert, for instance, a great deal of influence on such non-verbal issues as social distance, there exists a wide variety of acceptable behaviour within any culture. As a result, non-verbal behaviour is difficult to either quantify or to offer prescriptions about. Nevertheless, anyone who has met people with truly poor social skills can readily identify deviations from the norms of eye contact, distance, touch, verbal-turn-taking, posture and gesture. Therefore, these norms, however ephemeral, have meaning for us, and we respond accordingly when they are breached.

In the interview, responses to non-verbal cues may be based on the principle of 'watch, ask and act'. Thus, the nurse *watches* each of the broad constellations of non-verbal behaviour mentioned above, checking them against her own personal store of norms. She then *asks* herself what breaches of these norms mean for the client. For example:

'Is the client who is now avoiding eye contact ashamed of what she has just said? Trying to keep control by lowering her level of social contact? Shutting me out so that I don't ask her a question about this topic because it's so painful? Hiding tears? Exhausted?'

and so on. The interviewer may have other contextual evidence (both non-verbal and verbal) to support her ideas. The nurse then *acts* accordingly. Part of this action concerns the interviewer's own non-verbal behaviour, and here we are again in the realm of either inhibiting the interaction or of facilitating it through the use of reinforcing behaviours. Ideally the nurse uses non-verbal cues from the client to increase her awareness of the client's emotional state, and to offer a series of non-verbal behaviours which combine with her words effectively to convey understanding of that emotional state and encourage the client to express it further.

Thus, the nurse uses *eye contact* to convey interest, by concentrating on the client when she is talking, seeks a *distance* from the client where both are reasonably comfortable and convey that comfort by not seeking to alter the distance, generally maintains an attentive, still *posture* but mirrors the client's posture and *gestures* during times of particularly emotional communication by the client.

Touch is a particularly powerful aspect of non-verbal communication, and so deserves careful consideration by the interviewer (Weiss, 1979). Some years ago, I regularly showed a video of an interview to groups of nurses, and the aspect of the tape which caused most heated comment was when the interviewer touched the client's shoulder. Almost all the groups I showed the tape to were worried by the possibility of misinterpretation of touch, and by the acceptability of it to the client. A further concern, related to misinterpretation, was the fear of over-involvement. Much later, when preparing a reading list for students concerning non-verbal communication, I briefly reviewed many books, and was surprised to discover only *three* which even mentioned touch, and of these only one discussed its role in nurse–client interactions during offering of support in an interview (Sundeen *et al.*, 1989). This is particularly strange given that we know how powerful touch can be, and given that other aspects of nursing involve a great deal of touch, and some models of nursing even advocate the use of therapeutic touch as an intervention in its own right (Rogers, 1980).

Nevertheless, it would be strange if interviewers did not *want* to touch their clients, as part of offering solace and support. Thus, I offer the following suggestions regarding touch.

Bear in mind the 'assumptions about the client' made in Chapter 1, and trust the client.
Be guided by the client. Move closer and touch slowly at first. Observe the client's reactions throughout, and react accordingly.
Recognize that we, as interviewers, have needs and fears. Confront the fear of rejection by the client, and *test out* whether the client seeks touch.

The appropriate use of these non-verbal behaviours and the ability to read them in others are fairly basic social skills, which most humans acquire without special tuition, through social learning. It is important, therefore, not to apply them mechanically in interactions with clients. In the interview setting, stress may result in the use of these skills being diminished, both for interviewers and clients. Paying attention to appropriate non-verbal behaviour is, for most nurse interviewers, a question of reinstating, in the stressful situation of the interview, what is already present at other times. This may appear unnatural to the interviewer at first, but can soon become part of one's interviewing repertoire in the same way that it forms part of the social repertoire of most people. The same is true of the series of verbal facilitations of client support, exploration and consolation we will now examine. Many of these are aspects of everyday conversation which we simply need to reinstate into our clinical repertoire in order to be successful in facilitating clients. For this reason, we will draw our examples from ordinary social conversation rather than from clinical interviewing.

PARAPHRASING

In Chapter 5, we spoke about how reinforcement serves to increase a client's discussion of a particular topic, whilst summarizing offers the opportunity to check our understanding of what is being said and demonstrates our attention. Paraphrasing acts in the same ways, but is much briefer than the summary, repeating the theme contained in one or a few remarks by the client. The paraphrase is characterized by this emphasis on *theme* rather than content, aiming to demonstrate that the interviewer understands the significance of the client's words, rather than simply that she has been hearing them. In this way, paraphrasing differs from restatement, which is the simple reiteration of the client's actual words. This is, in itself, a useful tactic, but lacks the ability to convey *depth* of understanding in the way that paraphrasing does. The ability to tease out themes and trends is a key characteristic of active, facilitative listening. Here, two students are discussing an examination one of them has just taken.

Simon: It was terrible. I got into the exam and didn't know a thing on the paper. I couldn't believe it.

Andy: Really?

Simon: All this stuff came up about transcultural aspects of health. I was gutted!

Andy: Gutted, yeah. (*Restatement.*)

Simon: So anyway, I just sat there, and wrote the first things that came into my head.

Andy: It sounds like you had no idea what to put on the paper. (*Paraphrase.*)

Notice that Andy does not *interpret* what Simon says according to any theoretical view, but simply repeats the thematic content (being confused, at a loss) neither adding to nor subtracting from its meaning.

REFLECTING

Reflection goes one step beyond paraphrasing, by attempting, whilst demonstrating attentiveness, to guide the client further into the emotional aspects of her discourse. Again, the element of validating the client's attempts to examine her feelings is present, through the reinforcing properties of attention. Additionally, the interviewer attempts to assist the client in recognizing feelings which are expressed indirectly, thus reinforcing direct statement emotions and confrontation of them.

Simon: When I think of all the hours I put into looking at the legislation on health provision, social care and public health

Andy: You feel angry about all the wasted time. (*Reflection.*)

This is, I think, an accurate reflection on Andy's part, but does also bring to light an issue regarding reflection. Reflecting is a *kind* of interpretation of a client's remarks, and so the sensitive interviewer needs to consider carefully, before reflecting, whether or not the client would, in fact, have arrived at such a reflection without assistance. Often this is so, and in such cases, reflection by the interviewer is clumsy, disrupts the flow of the client's account, and misses the opportunity for the client to learn something unaided. By contrast, however, the well-timed reflection, particularly where it reveals to the client an emotion of which they had limited awareness, or reveals a conflict of emotions, can be extremely supportive and facilitative of the client's own investigations.

Since humans generally experience similar reactions to similar general stimuli, as a consequence of their common genetic inheritance and broad social background, it is reasonable for the interviewer to assume that aspects of the client's non-verbal communication indicate particular emotional states, and to reflect upon these also, yet here again it must be emphasized that, if emotions are being expressed non-verbally with any degree of force, they are likely to be as obvious to the client as to the interviewer, and so verbal reflection may well be intrusive and irrelevant.

CLARIFYING

Clarifying can refer to two separate kinds of interviewer behaviour. In the first, the interviewer seeks to clarify some issue for the client of which she is only vaguely aware. In this sense of the word, it is similar to paraphrasing, but involves broader, more general aspects of the client's meaning. In its second sense, the interviewer *seeks* clarification from the client about her meaning. As well as indicating her desire to understand and help the client, this tactic also offers the client the opportunity to restate her thoughts and feelings. This in itself may be helpful, by causing the client to examine them again.

Andy: Sorry, have I got this right? You were mainly fed up because of all the wasted time?

CONFRONTING

Confronting as a tactic is something which many interviewers are shy of, and for good reason. We are all aware that confrontation in many contexts has connotations of judgement, and interviewers are often taught to avoid judgement of the client. Furthermore, confrontation has overtones of aggression, a quality not generally associated with therapeutic change. Nevertheless, people *do* behave inappropriately, cover up things which frighten them, avoid issues. In real-life conversations outside the interview, we routinely challenge people outside interview settings about these behaviours, with more or less skill and more or less effect on their behaviour.

Effective confrontation in interviewing is almost always either feedback about the client's behaviour, feedback about our assumption about this behaviour or feedback about its effect upon us. In all these cases, the interviewer seeks to avoid judgement of the client, avoid the generation of hostility in the client consequent upon judgement, offer the client a learning experience and help the client to seek coping tactics. In offering feedback about behaviour, the interviewer will generally begin by *describing* it, in much the same as she would as part of a summary in assessment interviewing, possibly going even so far as to use an ABC approach. This emphasizes to the client that it is the *behaviour* that is being evaluated here, *not* the person. She then offers an *inference* about the meaning to the client of that behaviour and seeks clarification about the appropriateness of that inference.

Andy: During the run up to exams, you spent a lot of time looking at only a few aspects of the course, and never looked at stuff from the lectures you had missed. (*Description of behaviour.*) I think this was because you were actually put off from studying that stuff because of the amount of work it would have taken to get it up to scratch. (*Inference.*) What do you reckon? (*Seeking clarification about inference.*)

Feedback about the effect of a client's behaviour on us follows the statement of the behaviour with a simple statement of how this behaviour makes us feel. Feedback is then sought from the client about how it feels to know the effect her behaviour has on us.

Andy: Well, from the way you talk about what was on the paper (*Description of behaviour.*) I start to worry about whether I have done enough for my own exam tomorrow. (*Statement of feeling.*) That's the effect it has on me! (*Seeking feedback.*)

As you can see, confrontation again contains aspects of interpretation. In addition, it is potentially powerful because it brings the client face to face with her own behaviour and its effect on others. As with reflection, confrontation is a strong spice, and should be used sparingly and with discretion.

SELF-DISCLOSURE

In a sense, self-disclosure, where the interviewer reveals part of her own personality or history to the interviewee is a kind of confrontation, since it poses a certain threat to the interviewee, who is offered the experiences of the interviewer as a possible source of modelling for her own emotional investigation and coping. Like other forms of confrontation, it should be used with care. We are familiar with well-meaning people who offer copious examples, from their own experience, of advice which we might follow, and equally familiar with offers to share their suffering. Such excesses are inappropriate to the supportive interview, since they fail to address the uniqueness of the client's experience. Since no two people have had the same experiences, how can one's have relevance to the other's?

However, clients do find self-disclosure facilitative in some situations (Brammer *et al.*, 1988), provided it is relevant, limited and focal, for the following reasons:

Self-disclosure gives permission for having and expressing feelings.
Self-disclosure models how to express feelings.
Self-disclosure models coping with feelings.
Self-disclosure models coping with the expression of feelings.

In view of this, it is suggested that the earlier remarks about deciding when it is appropriate to touch the client also be followed with regard to self-disclosure.

REDIRECTING, QUESTIONING, SUMMARIZING

We encountered these three tactics during Chapter 5, and I suggested a rereading of parts of this chapter earlier. Apart from their importance in the context of information-gathering, and in reinforcing the client's contributions, redirecting, questioning and summarizing are also important in the facilitation of emotions. Like clarification, redirecting and questioning using primarily open questions both help to *focus* the client on the material under examination. This is just as true with emotional as with factual information. Important additional messages for the client are: (a) the importance of continuing confrontation of the difficult material (clients may seek to avoid it because of its anxiety-provoking nature); (b) that the interviewer is ready and willing to examine such material with the client (clients may believe that the interviewer will be uninterested or embarrassed, and interviewers themselves may seek to avoid such information, because of the anxiety it evokes in them); and (c) that the interviewer will assist them in examining and coping with that information (by redirecting them if they wander away from it, or summarizing in order to show attention and understanding).

In the context of facilitating emotion, summarizing is similar to paraphrasing in that it demonstrates the interviewer's understanding and offers the opportunity for correction of misconceptions regarding the meaning of the client's discourse. Unlike paraphrases, however, they refer to a number of client statements, and offer a precis of these, generally towards the end of a theme. The interviewer can also use summarizing as a way of controlling the flow of the interview. For example, the interviewer may summarize in order to bring a particular aspect of the interview to a close, and then move the client on, or to draw an interview to a close, avoiding starting on new issues late on in the interaction.

Andy: Yeah, I think I can see now how you spent such a lot of time revising one area, and were really fed up when it didn't come up on the paper. Have you any idea what to do now? (*Summary with redirection.*)

RELAXING

We mentioned relaxation in Chapter 3, as a tactic that might help interviewers to reflect. It is worth mentioning here, however, that relaxation can also help the client who feels exhausted or overcome by the emotions which have been explored during a session. Relaxation does not itself help the client to come to terms with emotions, what the interviewer here offers is some time off from thinking about such issues when they become too difficult, and demonstration to the client that emotions need not overwhelm her, since short-term relief, at least, is possible.

REASSURANCE

Rarely in the nursing literature has so complex a topic been dealt with so poorly, or in so many diverse ways. In nursing in hospital and other medical settings, all commentators seem to be united in agreeing that reassurance is a key nursing role: on admission, before a difficult procedure, after return from surgery, prior to discharge, and so on. Yet how does the nurse go about reassuring a client, and under what circumstances is it appropriate to do so?

A key concept about reassurance is that it operates, at least according to cognitive-behaviourists, according to the rules governing reward and punishment. In certain circumstances, reassurance is either reinforcing or punishing. Thus two fundamental rules emerge for the nurse:

Avoid using reassurance as punishment.
When using reassurance as reinforcement, be sure you know what behaviours, thoughts and feelings you are reinforcing.

Since the notion that reassurance can be punishing is a counter-intuitive notion, let's examine this first. First, it should be noted that the term 'punishment' is used without any evaluative connotations. Instead, I have retained the traditional behavioural definition of punishment we touched on in Chapter 4 – the withdrawal of a reward or the application of an aversive stimulus, with the result that the particular behaviour to which the punishment is applied tends to decrease in frequency. In this sense of the word we routinely punish the activities of others as part of our daily interactions. For instance, we regulate conversation by averting gaze, thus withdrawing the reinforcement of attention. Likewise, when we show anger towards someone because of their behaviour, we punish them by causing the occurrence of the aversive stimulus of autonomic arousal (as in fear or guilt) within them. Cognitive-behaviourists make no statement about whether or not we *should* behave in this way, other than to note that punishment is seldom an effective tactic in changing behaviour. Its effectiveness in situations such as the ones I have just outlined is generally because of reinforcement of activities other than the ones being punished.

To return, then, to the notion of reassurance as punishment, consider the following situation:

Client: I find the prospect of surgery very worrying.

Nurse: Don't worry, Doctor Smith is a very good surgeon.

This seems straightforward enough. Here, the clinician punishes the client by differential withdrawal of attention from the aspect of importance to the client – in this case, 'being worried', and attends only to the procedural aspect of the sentence. Effectively, the nurse's communication here is: 'talk to me about facts, not about feelings', thus punishing the client's emotional expression and rendering it less likely to occur on subsequent occasions. However, the message is, in fact, conveyed even more forcefully than this, since there is a further punishment embedded in the nurse's reply. The words don't worry represent a negation of the client's experience of 'being worried', rendering such concerns invalid, as a rule, as well as of no interest to the nurse on this occasion. General expressions like 'don't worry', 'it will be all right', 'there's nothing to worry about', and so on, are all examples of this covert punishment in the guise of reassurance.

However, even very explicit information which attempts to reassure the client can, in fact, be punishing. The offering of even highly specific procedural information to a client who in fact requires an opportunity to voice her own fears about the forthcoming procedure is punishing. Indeed, the more such information is offered in such inappropriate situations, the more punishing it is likely to become, as the client experiences the nurse ignoring her concerns and invalidating their importance to an even greater degree.

As an alternative tactic, the skilful interviewer allows herself to be led by the client in such situations, relying on paraphrasing and reflection to express concern and empathy for the client and open questions and statements to allow the client to specify when, whether and what information is required as part of the reassurative process. With regard to the offering of such information, the principle of orientating the client, which we discussed in Chapter 5, is a good guideline to the effective delivery of reassuring information.

Turning now to the idea of reassurance as reinforcement, the first thing to note is that we will often want to use reassurance in just this way. Principally, this will be the case when clients are seeking reassurance about their own performance.

Indeed, it may well be that the seeking of such reassurance represents a failure on our own parts as nurses, since we should have become adept at offering plentiful reinforcement, as part of our role in facilitation of client performance and supporting the client during the undertaking of therapeutic instructions. In this situation, the most appropriate form of reassurance to the client is the application of *accurate feedback* about performance. In the following example, the client is unsure about whether she has been following therapeutic instructions accurately.

Client: Yes, that idea you gave me about putting a wedge under my bottom when sitting in front of the VDU. I've tried it, but I'm not sure I'm doing it right. (*Gives description.*)

Nurse: Most of this seems fine. (*General reinforcement.*) The wedge you're using is about the right height, and it seems to be helping you to keep your back straight. (*Specific positive feedback on performance.*) Mind you, you don't seem to be using the wedge every time you work at the VDU. (*Specific negative feedback on performance.*) Is there some way in which we can fix that? (*Opening negotiation about alternative coping tactic.*)

Towards the end of the interchange, the nurse offers some negative feedback about difficulties with the client's performance. It is now well recognized that people can benefit from negative as well as positive feedback (Welford, 1976), but it is equally clear that the maximum benefit is to be derived from such feedback if it is delivered in the context of positive feedback about other elements of performance and positive reinforcement for attempts at performance. More-over, it is of comparatively little use to deliver such feedback in the absence of some attempt to introduce alternative tactics which the client can use, as the nurse does at the end of this example this example.

In general, reassurance is least problematic when it is reinforcing in the ways described in the above example. In this interaction, the nurse deliberately rein-forces only those actions which are associated either with the client's attempts at coping or with positive outcomes from treatment, much as we suggested in Chapter 5. As well as offering reassurance regarding the appropriateness of the activities to be performed, the sensitive nurse also encourages the *act* of seeking reassurance about such matters, since it is a valuable source of information about the client's compliance, and a useful opportunity to correct misconceptions and renegotiate problematic instructions. Such requests for reassurance about the nature of treatment can, however, themselves become part of the problem, as the client and nurse both become preoccupied with this process of reassurance rather than the process of coping with the client's difficulties, as in this example of a client with fears about illness:

Client: I had a lot of difficulty over the past week, because I knew we'd agreed that I would not phone my doctor except in a dire emergency, and we'd agreed that only chest pain different from what I have usually had would

> count. But I couldn't decide about several episodes, and so I didn't contact him. Was that OK?

Nurse: Yes, that's fine, and I think it was really good that you managed to resist the urge to phone your GP. Tell me, did anything awful happen as a result?

Client: No!

Superficially, the above response by the nurse seems to fit the bill rather well. It combines affirmation of the what client has said with specific reinforcement of the contracted behaviour (not telephoning the GP) and an invitation to the client to examine the way she has been able to test her fears against reality. However, the difficulty here is that part of the client's problem is about risk-taking, and this is itself being mirrored in being unable to take risks about the nature of treatment, and thus needing to check out even quite minute areas of doubt. Since we know that people with illness fears share a number of characteristics with people with problems of compulsive checking (Salkovskis & Warwick, 1986), a complete cognitive-behavioural response addresses the issue of the need for certainty with regard to the here-and-now of the therapeutic interaction, as well as the situation described by the client in seeking clarification:

Nurse: I think it was excellent that you managed to stop yourself from contacting the GP (*Reinforcement of coping tactic.*), but it's impossible for me to tell you whether you made the right choice in discriminating between these episodes and your usual chest pain. Perhaps you can tell *me* whether you think you made the right choice? (*Emphasizing client responsibility.*)

In this variant, the nurse opens the way for the client to offer *herself* reassurance, by reflecting on her performance, and avoids becoming locked into a pattern of providing continuing validation of the client's quest for a resolution to her uncertainties. Clearly, there are some situations where such a quest is highly valid, and the nurse's responsibility is primarily to elicit those areas of doubt and difficulty and respond to them with the offer of appropriate information. In this case, however, as in many health care interactions, the issue is that there are no definitive 'answers'. In such situations, the nurse is involved in frank discussion of the inevitability of uncertainty for the client, the effect that has on the client in terms of anxiety, and what tactics (such as the negotiation of a *ban* on reassurance-seeking in the case of the client discussed here and her GP) will help the client to cope with such anxiety.

The issue of inappropriate reassurance-giving is perhaps seen at its most problematic when the clinician mistakes the reinforcing nature of reassurance to such a degree that she comes to reinforce *only* the act of reassurance-seeking. In cognitive-behavioural terms, the main flaw in such a policy is its total lack of effectiveness in decreasing client anxiety, together with its tendency to increase the number of occasions on which reassurance is sought. Since almost all nursing models share with cognitive-behavioural formulations of client distress the aim of promoting the maximum client independence possible, this latter problem represents a formidable difficulty, being completely at odds with such an aim. According to the cognitive-behavioural account, lack of awareness of what is being reinforced leads to offering powerful rewards for the seeking of reassurance, rather than for coping with difficulties or seeking advice regarding coping. If a nurse enables a client to feel less anxious about a procedure, a problem, or the future in general, without offering some concrete coping tactic which the client herself can use, this is simply a fostering of dependence. The client comes to associate the nurse's presence, and perhaps certain verbal forms she uses (e.g. 'Don't worry', ' It will be OK', 'It will soon be over', 'Don't be silly') with feelings of decreased anxiety. Although it is part of the nurse's role to decrease anxiety, the advantage of this upon a single occasion has to be weighed against the possible disadvantages in the long term, whether that be on subsequent interactions with this nurse, with other nurses, on subsequent admissions or during subsequent problematic episodes. In the situation described here, the client has learnt nothing about coping with anxiety other than that the presence of the nurse serves as an anxiety reducer. According to operant conditioning theory, we cannot therefore expect a diminution of client anxiety on subsequent occasions of threat, since she has not experienced independent coping and anxiety reduction, only anxiety reduction as a consequence of seeking reassurance from another. Thus, the only likely change for the client will be an increase in the number of occasions on which reassurance is sought, as the client seeks a reduction in anxiety symptoms in the only way which has been demonstrated to be effective.

In the light of this, we have further reason to be abundantly clear about what kinds of client behaviour we are reinforcing when we offer verbal reassurance of this 'blanket' kind. It may be helpful, then, to break down the original two rules of reassurance (avoid punishment and take care what you reinforce) as follows:

Reinforce client coping attempts.
Reinforce client behaviours associated with positive outcomes.
Discriminate between requests for reassurative information and expressions of anxiety and respond accordingly.
Encourage examination of repeated requests for reassurance.
Avoid reinforcement (through temporary anxiety reduction by the nurse without the offer of coping tactics or information) of requests for reassurance rather than coping.
Encourage the client to self-reassure through the use of exploration of client statements and actions.

MANAGING TIME IN THE SUPPORTIVE INTERVIEW AND THE USE OF EXPOSURE

All the tactics we have examined in this chapter are, in one way or another, about giving the client *time* to explore and possibly to come to terms with their emotions. Likewise, all these tactics involve the nurse in staying out of the client's way, and facilitating her in exploring these emotional aspects of her difficulties. Naturally, support is a requirement in almost *all* interviews, but some difficulties require a *primarily* supportive approach. These supportive interviews are characterized, in general, by openness of questioning or by the utterance of statements which promote the flow of the client's discourse about her feelings and her experience of them. In this sense, then, supportive interviews are amongst the most client-led that skilled interviewers conduct. Nevertheless, the interviewer does attempt to guide the client, through the use of the tactics we have described, towards a fuller understanding and confrontation of emotional issues, and is, in this sense, highly active.

Exposure

For cognitive-behaviourists, part of this process involves the client in ceasing to escape from previously avoided material and its emotional effects, in just the same way that phobics are advised to confront previously avoided situations and behaviours, using the now-familiar argument that confrontation leads to a diminution of anxiety. It is well-documented that this process succeeds best with long and frequent contact with the frightening stimulus. With this in mind, all the tactics described in this chapter become seen as ways of keeping the client in contact with her emotions for sufficiently long for this diminution to occur. Verbalizing the painful material is, in this sense, a kind of exposure treatment (Marks, 1987), which decreases the ability of the problematic material to give rise to the unwanted emotional response. In addition to straightforward verbal description, the interviewer can encourage the client to imagine the situations as she is describing them, and describe them as though they were happening in the here-and-now, repeatedly, until anxiety reduction comes about.

Most important in this process of exposure is the ending of contact: in this case, the supportive phase of an interview. The skilful interviewer ensures that the client has enough time to pursue the difficult topics as much as she wants, and ensures that the interview ends at a point when some anxiety-reduction has taken place. Both these issues require the interviewer to be acutely aware of the passage of time in the interview, and to manage that time in such a way that these two objectives are met. This is difficult, but of considerable importance, since to leave the client without anxiety reduction at the end of an interview of this kind lets pass the opportunity for the client to learn about coping, and reinforces patterns of avoidant emotional responding associated with continuing difficulty. It is also problematic from the point of view of intervention, since the interviewer thus comes to be associated with the arousal of unpleasant feelings, but not with their cessation, and may, therefore, become an anxiety-provoking stimulus herself. In view of this, the interviewer needs to regulate the flow of emotional material by encouraging the client to bring forth such material sufficiently early in the interview to allow as much examination of it as possible, and to resist attempts to bring forward such information late in the interview. It is natural to wish to avoid painful experiences, and to attempt to curtail the amount of time spent in discussion of them. Clients who do this need to know (a) that the interviewer is willing to discuss the material with them, (b) that the interviewer understands that the material is painful, and (c) that the interviewer understands that the material needs more time than is available at the end of an interview. In the light of these three conditions, most clients will accept redirection of such material to the beginning of the next session. It is almost always a mistake to prolong an interview to take account of information introduced late on, however tempting this may be. Cognitive-behaviourists tend *not* to accept one common interpretation of such 'late' material – the manipulation and testing of the clinician by the client. There are, however, several *other* reasons for avoiding prolongation of the interview. First, such an action rewards with attention the client's introduction of such material, and it is as well to avoid this, since this encourages the client to do so again, introducing the possibility that such information will always be dealt with in a rushed way. Second, the interviewer often has other clients waiting! As well as being disrespectful to them, it is unlikely that the interviewer can give her full attention to her current client if half her mind is concerned with closing the session so as to see the next. Finally, the client may have introduced the information late precisely because she felt unable to cope with a long examination of it. Here, the best course of action for the sensitive interviewer is to introduce this possibility, as part of examining the material during the next interview.

For appropriate handling of time in supportive interviewing, then, the following principles may be useful:

Never hurry the client (we as nurses also sometimes want to avoid painful material!).
Allow sufficient time for some degree of anxiety reduction.
Help the client to focus on small enough aspects of painful material for anxiety reduction to be practical in the given time.
Discourage the introduction of new material late in an interview.
Avoid extending the duration of a session to accommodate late information.

CLINICAL EXAMPLE

Here, David, a cancer support nurse, talks with Mr Adams about the recent death of his wife. The pair have met on one previous occasion, for assessment. We join the interview after some time has passed, and Mr Adams is discussing the funeral.

Mr A: The thing about it was, it was all so clinical. It didn't feel like it was her at all . . .

David: It didn't feel like it was her. (*Restatement.*)

Mr A: No, it was just like any other funeral. I've had lots of friends die over the years, and I suppose I always knew Maisie would die before I did, but when it came to it, it just didn't seem like it was happening.

David: In spite of all the preparation, you still weren't prepared. (*Para-phrasing*.)

Mr A: I don't think you ever are, are you, no matter how you try and accept the inevitable. You keep on hoping, and then there you are, listening to the priest and all that carry on.

David: You felt it had no meaning. (*Reflection*.)

Mr A: None at all, and I'm a religious man, always had a strong faith.

David: But now? (*Clarifying*.)

Mr A: Well, I feel as if I've lost my faith. I mean, you see people in the street, and you just even wish . . .

David: Even wish . . . (*Confronting through repetition*.)

Mr A: Well, you wish it was them and not her. It's hard to believe until you go through it.

David: I have never lost anyone close to me, but I think I get some impression from you of how awful it is. (*Self-disclosure and feedback of effect of client's words*.) Like nothing in the past could prepare you for it. (*Testing inference*.)

Mr A: Yes, quite dreadful.

David: You were telling me about what happened on the day of the funeral. (*Redirecting and encouraging confrontation of painful material*.)

The interview continues, and Mr Adams repeatedly examines the theme of isolation and disbelief. David summarizes.

David: We've talked a good deal about the funeral, and the main thing that's come over has been your feeling of disbelief, almost as though you were trying to make it all not have happened? (*Seeking feedback on inference*.)

Mr A: Yes, that's how it seems to me talking about it now.

David: That was the feeling I got from you. Well, there are about 10 minutes left before the end of our session, and I think we ought to leave things here, because we couldn't really talk enough about a new issue, and we seem to have come to a natural pause. Can we use these next minutes to discuss how the session has gone, and to think about how we'll follow on when we meet next time. (*Managing time to ensure anxiety reduction at the end of the session. Planning*.)

Once again, this case example is highly condensed, to include as many of the relevant points as possible. It is particularly important, with the exploratory, supportive interview, to note that a real interview would contain *far fewer* interviewer comments in this much time. Interviewers differ considerably in the amount they intervene, and it is important not to apply the suggestions here mechanically. The following exercises may help to avoid this.

EXERCISES

1 Over the next week, spend 10 minutes each day observing social conversations, noting each of the aspects of non-verbal behaviour described above. Spend another 10 minutes just noting occurrences of the facilitative verbal remarks we have examined.

2 Using the reflective techniques we examined in Chapter 3, examine the following

a very happy incident in your past,
a very sad one.

Consider how you would disclose each incident to a client, in order to help them exploring their own difficulties, and consider how much you would disclose in each case.

3 In your interactions with clients, focus on each of the facilitative verbal behaviours in turn, and examine its effect on the client, using the reflective techniques. Naturally, you will be using a great many skills at once, but *examine* only one on any occasion. Consider how you used it, and how to improve upon your performance.

4 Although the structure of the supportive interview seems loose, it is still present. Examine this structure by using the content of this chapter to arrive at a series of aims and objectives for the supportive interview.

5 Devise a protocol to help a client learn a *simple* relaxation exercise. Start with Jacobson's (1938) muscular relaxation and modify it to make it more simply carried out. Investigate the use of breathing exercises as relaxation (Salkovskis *et al.*, 1986).

FURTHER READING

Argyle, M. (1988) *Bodily Communication*. London. Routledge.
Brammer, L.M. (1988) *The Helping Relationship. Process and Skills*. Englewood Cliffs, NJ. Prentice Hall.
Trower, P. Bryant, B. & Argyle, M. (1978) *Social Skills and Mental Health*. London. Methuen.

8 Evaluating interventions

THE NATURE OF THE EVALUATIVE PROCESS

During our discussion of client assessment, we examined the notion of setting intervention goals with the client, and noted that this process also formed an introduction, for the client, to the idea of measurement and evaluation of her difficulties. This kind of evaluation, using measures, is a very formal and, in some ways, artificial process. Nevertheless, *all* evaluation, however informal, involves measurement, since, even if we simply ask the client whether they now feel better or worse than previously, we are requesting a judgement of the comparative magnitude of their difficulties (Yule & Helmsley, 1977). This is no different from asking if you prefer peaches or plums. In responding, some internal scale – 'liking' – is consulted for both peaches and plums, and 'scores' on the liking scale are recorded. The item that 'scores' higher is liked more. So, it may be that the artificiality of formal numerical measurement is more apparent than real.

In Chapter 5, we touched on the idea of interim target setting, and discussed this further in the chapter concerning education and advice. We now return to the kinds of goals that occupied most of our time in Chapter 5, those concerning eventual treatment outcome. The gathering of this quantitative baseline information is the crucial first step in detailed evaluation, and also gets the client thinking in an evaluative way.

WHEN TO EVALUATE

As may be inferred from the previous paragraph, there are some senses in which evaluation is clearly a continuous process, commencing at assessment. There is certainly no doubt that clients will evaluate their progress continuously, and nurses may do so also. There are, however, difficulties associated with too frequent evaluation. Nurse and client may become too involved in the minutiae of intervention by, for example, attempting to draw conclusions about outcome from client performance on specific interim goals. We noted in Chapter 6 that consideration of interim goals should *relate* them to long-term aims, but attempting to evaluate the latter through performance on the former alone should be avoided. Associated with this overemphasis on short-term goals may be a tendency to catastrophize minor setbacks which are a part of most interventions, owing to the unrealistic expectations and needs of both client and nurse. This may be particularly problematic if it occurs in the early stages of intervention, when other successes have not yet occurred, and the nurse–client relationship is also less robust than will (hopefully) be the case later in the intervention. Furthermore, repeated evaluations may be a sign of lack of confidence in the client on the part of the nurse. This in turn may communicate itself to the client, to the detriment of their relationship, and of compliance with the interventions they have negotiated. Finally, repeated evaluation does not empower the client, since it places undue emphasis on the nurse's role in controlling the process of treatment. One important aspect of written evaluation which is often overlooked is its function in formalizing the process and, therefore, increasing its salience, reminding both client and clinician of the difficulties associated with over-frequent evaluation.

As a general rule, then, frequent evaluations should be reserved for evaluation of the *process* of the intervention and its short-term, interim targets. Formal, written assessments of client progress by client and nurse, by contrast, will happen relatively infrequently, occurring at the beginning and end of treatment, and at previously negotiated and agreed points during the course of the intervention (Marks, 1986).

Leaving aside the initial, baseline evaluation, which is an evaluation of the client's own efforts prior to seeking treatment, rather than of the intervention itself, the selection of the formal evaluation points suggested here has several advantages, over and above the avoidance of the difficulties of over-frequent evaluation mentioned above. Since client and interviewer have negotiated evaluation points in advance, they have implicitly made a contract to give each particular intervention tactic, and, indeed, their therapeutic liaison as a whole, a *fair trial*. This in itself involves commitment, and may, therefore, be facilitative of the intervention. Equally, they have implicitly agreed that there may be setbacks during treatment, but that these will not alone constitute a failure in treatment. It may be necessary to review the process of intervention, particularly in the light of new information becoming available, but not the general rationale. As an example, a client with chronic back pain may, during the course of our interventions, suffer some acute exacerbation as a result of traumatic injury to the back. Clearly this will affect the conduct of our intervention, perhaps indicating slowing down, allowing time for the injury to resolve or for physiotherapy to be effective, but will not give rise to changes in our proposed general rationale for treatment of the chronic pain.

A third agreement implicit in the contracting of specific evaluation points is that treatment will, in fact, have an end. In this way, client and interviewer reduce the likelihood of dependence upon each other growing during the course of treatment (see Haley, 1969, for an ironical but important discussion of how therapists foster dependence to the detriment of their clients). All these three implicit agreements will almost certainly be stated *explicitly* during the assessment phase of treatment. Building them into the evaluative process offers an additional reinforcement of these messages for the client.

A further advantage of fixed-point evaluation is the avoidance of bias. We have already described the danger implicit in evaluating immediately after a treatment setback. The opposite, evaluating after a particularly successful session, is also problematic, since client and nurse may gain a mistaken view of how effective treatment has been. A major additional problem is the unconscious use of evaluation as a way of terminating treatment. We may well want to do such a thing consciously, and if this is so contracted between nurse and client, this is fair enough, but difficulty arises if either nurse or client or both do so without awareness. Thus, the nurse or client may ask for evaluation after a particular high or low point, and use the result, although atypical, as a rationale for termination. The nurse or client may also ask for evaluation at such times as a way of seeking reinforcement or reassurance. This is all quite legitimate, but is better examined in an open agenda. The use of fixed-point evaluation reduces the likelihood of use of evaluation in a biased way, since the evaluation points are fixed in advance, and the results gained from them are thus more likely to be representative of the client's progress in general (Marks, 1986).

Although I have outlined numerous advantages to formal, numerical evaluation of outcome goals at fixed points during intervention, there are also disadvantages to this system. The most important of these is lack of flexibility. Whilst it is important to give interventions a fair trial, and to recognize the distinction between making changes to the process of treatment and attempting to change its whole focus and rationale, there is also no doubt that clients' goals *do* shift during the course of treatment, sometimes voluntarily, and sometimes because of circumstances beyond their control. If used inflexibly, fixed-point evaluation cannot cope with shifting client needs and life-goals. However, if client and nurse are working together effectively, and, in particular, if the nurse is interviewing in the ways we have examined earlier, maximizing client power in the interview, it is possible to identify these shifts in client needs during *informal* evaluation, and to negotiate new outcome goals accordingly (Kazdin, 1982). Caution is needed here, however, since the desire to negotiate new goals may spring from dissatisfaction with the progress of the intervention, rather than with changing needs. If this is so, it is the dissatisfaction and the intervention which need to be the subject of examination, not the goals. A client's assertion that previously set goals are now seen as too difficult should be treated with the same caution. It may well be that such goals need renegotiating, but this should be the last consideration, after examining whether changes in the process of intervention might facilitate achievement of the goals which both client and nurse originally felt were appropriate.

A second disadvantage of fixed-point evaluation lies in deciding when these points should occur. Formal evaluation is a potentially profound source of reinforcement for the client, but also a potential source of punishment, if no progress appears to be being made. Successful interviewers will want to maximize the chances of reinforcement occurring, and minimize the likelihood of punishment. Thus, formal evaluation needs to be scheduled so that enough time has elapsed for improvement to be noticed, but *only just enough*, so that the opportunity for reinforcement is not delayed. When these points occur is dependent primarily on the nature of the client's difficulty and the experience and expertise of the nurse in judging the likely speed of client progress, and the range of possibilities is, therefore, potentially vast. In my own area, behavioural medicine, it might be appropriate to offer a client with motor tics a first intermediate formal evaluation after two or three sessions, since this difficulty characteristically responds very quickly (Azrin & Nunn, 1973), whilst a client attempting to learn to identify and modify the onset of epileptic seizures would be a much more complex proposition, since (a) the occurrence of the difficulty itself might be of highly variable frequency and (b) cognitive-behavioural interventions are in an early stage of development and predictions about treatment duration are, therefore, problematic, and frequent careful monitoring is required. It is possible, however, to arrive at general guidelines for the frequency of evaluation. Frequency is a function of *problem severity*, *known durations* of the treatment, *known efficacy* of treatment and *experience of the nurse* in offering the particular intervention. Thus, the more severe the difficulty, the longer it is likely to take for change to occur, if all the other elements held constant. Similarly, the more well-supported the effectiveness of the intervention, the less frequent the evaluation of outcome; the less experienced the clinician, the less frequent the evaluation (since less experienced clinicians can be expected to achieve results more slowly); the slower the intervention to work, the less frequent the evaluations. A combination of these factors allows us to present the client with a reasonable estimate of how often formal evaluation might occur, and the client herself can help by adding additional information about her own perception of problem severity, the amount of time she is able to devote to addressing it and how frequent she feels feedback of this kind needs to be.

HOW TO EVALUATE

In discussing frequency and organization of evaluation, we spoke of the risk of bias. This is also an issue in the *process* of the evaluation interview, either formal or informal. The avoidance of bias is a key issue in the process of evaluation (Peck & Shapiro, 1990). The interviewer can bias the evaluation process in three principle ways. Let us examine each in turn.

The interviewer has control over *when* evaluation takes place. As we have noted, this can be a source of bias by the interviewer's choosing a time during a course of treatment which is most favourable, but the interviewer may also choose to vary the point during a particular session at which evaluative elements are offered. Offering the opportunity for evaluation at the end of a successful session pretty well ensures an artificially inflated estimate of success by the client. The interviewer controls *the way* in which evaluative questioning occurs, and may choose words which either frame the client's problem in its most positive light, or openly lead the client towards a desired response. These 'demand characteristics' are a well-documented source of bias in a great many psychological variables (Orne, 1962). Finally, the interviewer controls *what* is evaluated, and may decide to ask questions which relate primarily to those areas where she knows treatment has been effective. By contrast, areas of less success may receive less emphasis in the evaluation process.

Measurement and the use of predetermined criteria for success reduce these dangers considerably (Kazdin, 1982). However, they remain present, even when using highly structured evaluation tools. It should not be supposed that the interviewer deliberately sets out to 'cook the books' of treatment outcome. Rather, bias is ever-present, and many of the elements which produce it are outside our awareness. Since clinicians want to be successful, and have a personal investment in success, it is reasonable to assume that their bias will tend to be in a positive direction, although no doubt some individuals, whether through scepticism about the treatment methods they are employing or lack of faith in their own abilities, will tend to bias results negatively. Equally, 'favoured' clients may be offered questions in a way which makes positive answers more likely, both since the clinician *wants* that client to be successful, because of personal investment in her, and because the clinician *believes* she has been more successful, because of the halo effect surrounding the client. Nor are clinicians alone in being subject to such biases. Clients are likely to bias their responses, both as a reaction to particular demand characteristics, but also owing to their own need to succeed and to please the clinician (Coolican, 1990).

As minimum tactics for decreasing bias in evaluations, the following procedures are recommended:

Ensure that evaluation, whether formal or informal, takes place at a regular, predetermined time in each session for which evaluation is scheduled.
Follow the written details of each target statement precisely during formal evaluation.
Describe the scales associated with the evaluation of each target on each occasion for evaluation.
Do not remind the client of previous scores until after completion of each evaluation.
Pay attention to tone of voice so as to avoid cuing the client to particular scores which you favour.
Show the client written targets and score-sheets wherever possible, and check for understanding of the scales repeatedly.
Follow precisely the guidelines in Chapter 5 for negotiation of target statements.
Use third party reports (relatives, friends, other clinicians) to corroborate the value of evaluative ratings wherever this is possible and has been agreed with the client.
Use written records of client achievements as corroboration wherever possible.

Two final considerations related to evaluation of a course of intervention concern the content of the evaluative material and the importance to be ascribed to the evaluative process. With regard to content, once again, the suggestions in Chapter 5 on target-setting should be followed, and will hopefully lead to comprehensiveness of coverage of those areas of concern to the client. It is important, however, that each formal evaluation (and indeed most informal evaluation) addresses each of the issues identified at assessment, not only to ensure unbiased reporting, but also to demonstrate to the client the importance of *her* view of her difficulties, since the interviewer refrains from censorship of any aspect of the difficulties. Secondly, evaluation is a crucial part of intervention, both for clinician and client, for reasons we discussed in Chapter 5. This importance should be reflected in the way the interviewer deals with evaluation. Therefore, evaluation should never be rushed. In the case of a client with complex diffi-culties, clinician and client may decide to set aside the whole of a session, or a number of sessions, just for evaluation. Even where the nature of both the problem and of intervention do not justify the expenditure of a whole interview on evaluation, there should be specific time earmarked within the interview for this activity, and this should be adequate for the task. Rushed evaluation conveys to the client the message that it is not valued by the clinician. If this is so, what does the clinician think about the client's difficulties, and why should the client value or commit to the evaluation process?

In the following example, Nina, a practice nurse, attempts to evaluate a client's negotiated goals of:

'Reduction of headache frequency from daily to once per fortnight'

and:

'Reduction of headache severity by 70%'

using mutually agreed percentage scales. It is the end of an agreed course of six sessions of relaxation training.

CLINICAL EXAMPLE

Nina: You remember, Jane, that when we first met, we agreed that our final evaluation would be during our last scheduled session, which is today? (*Fixed-point formal evaluation.*)

Jane: Yes.

Nina: Well, I have the scales we drew up together, and the goals which we agreed and which we also evaluated at the beginning of our third meeting. So as to be consistent, I'm going to suggest that we do it at the beginning of this session, too. (*Eliminating bias.*)

Jane: OK.

Nina: OK. Now, I'll just show you the goal statements again, along with the scale. (*Shows papers, but not previous scores, eliminating bias.*) You remember we agreed on percentage scales – a percentage success scale for the first goal, and a percentage pain scale for the second?

Jane: (Reads scales, nods, smiles.)

Nina: OK, so what do you think for the first target: 'Reduction of headache frequency from daily to once per fortnight'. Your percentage success in achieving that target? (*Monotonous, formal tone of voice, eliminating bias.*)

Jane: Well, on the basis of the last 2 weeks, I would have to say 90%

Nina: Excellent! (*Reinforcing attainment.*) Just to be clear, your saying you're 90% of the way towards achieving that target. (*Checking comprehension of scale.*)

Jane: Mmm.

Nina: And that would represent how many headaches in that fortnight? (*Checking validity of scale estimate for client.*)

Jane: Well, three, in fact, but two were very brief and mild.

Nina: OK, and you're happy to rate the improvement at 90%?

Jane: Definitely.

Nina: Thank you. Can we go on now to look at your second target.

> *Nina then examines this target, before seeking ratings from Jane of the effect more generally of improvement in the headaches on her life, both formally, through the use of further rating scales [perhaps of work, social and leisure aspects of the life (Marks, 1986)]. Only then does she offer feedback about previous scores, thus avoiding contamination of the current scores.*

Nina: Well, having a look back at your first ratings on goal 1, you actually rated no success at all in decreasing headache – 0 per cent, so your rating today of 90 per cent seems like a huge improvement, and bears out what you were saying about the effect on your life in general.

EXERCISES

1 In this chapter, you will notice that once again we did not examine aims and objectives for the evaluative interview. Using your knowledge of aims and objectives, and the examples in previous chapters, draw up a series of aims and objectives which the interviewer would hope to meet during the course of the evaluative interview.

2 Look back on the exercises associated with Chapter 5, and decide how you would go about checking client progress using the scales you devised.

3a If you are sufficiently far through an intervention with a client with whom you are using the evaluative techniques we have discussed in this book (including measurement), conduct the evaluative interview.

3b If you do not have a client this far through intervention, focus on the suggestions for effective evaluation in this chapter and apply them to your current methods of evaluation with a client you are working with who is nearing discharge.

FURTHER READING

Coolican, H. (1992) *Research Methods and Statistics in Psychology*. London. Hodder & Stoughton.
Peck, D.F. & Shapiro, C.M. (1990) *Measuring Human Problems: A Practical Guide*. Chichester. Wiley.

9 Ending a series of interviews

Many book chapters have been written about the nature of ending a series of therapeutic interactions with clients, and it is often considered that the termination phase of a relationship is one of the most difficult. Certainly, if we consider our informal personal relationships, there is no doubt that endings give rise to strong emotions, whether these involve grief, sadness, regret or even relief (Parkes, 1972). Throughout this book, we have stressed the importance of the role of the client as an active participant in the interviewing process, and the need for collaboration with her. Given the amount of involvement which we have advocated that the sensitive interviewer will have with the interviewee, it would seem logical to suppose that some of the feelings we have about ending informal relationships will also occur in the more formal setting of the interview, for both interviewer and client.

Nevertheless, this chapter is one of the briefest in the whole book. This is not because the importance of appropriate ending to a series of interviews is to be underestimated, but because, in cognitive-behavioural approaches to interviewing, the point of ending is implicitly worked towards from the beginning of the first interview, through the very process of involving the client in the process of interviewing and intervention, just as we have worked through to the closing of this book by introducing exercises, some of which have explicitly asked you to take over the construction of part of the book's content.

This process seeks to maximize client independence from the outset, and aims to define the roles of client and interviewer within the context of that independence. In cognitive-behavioural interviewing, the role of the nurse may well be one of adviser, supporter, listener, questioner or teacher. It is *never* one of friend. Although, as we have discussed, empathy and consideration for the client underpin much of the specific technical approach to interviewing embodied by the cognitive-behavioural approach, and this in itself demands a *friendly* approach to the client, sensitive interviewers are also sensitive to themselves, recognize their needs for the friendship and esteem of others, and take steps to minimize the likelihood of these needs intruding into the interview. The interviewing relationship is intrinsically different from friendship relationships because it is more focal in content, more limited in terms of time and setting and more circumscribed in terms of goals. Most important, the interview is a highly artificial setting, in which the motivations of the two participants differ greatly from those of people in less formal relationships, and in which the degree of power allotted to the participants is extremely skewed (Dillon, 1990). It seems unlikely that a relationship which differs so greatly from what we generally understand as friendship could ever be so misconstrued, yet therapists of all kinds *are* attracted to their clients in such ways, even to the extent of sexual intimacy (Masson, 1990). In the course of a very moving account of his personal approach to therapy, Arnold Lazarus (Dryden, 1991) describes how it is sometimes possible to break this rule about the establishment of (non-sexual) friendships with clients. However, most of us lack either the experience, sensitivity or expertise of an Arnold Lazarus, and so would be well-advised to continue to draw this distinction between friendly professional support and friendship. The kind of social distance the cognitive-behavioural interviewer seeks to created is that which typically occurs between a trusted teacher and gifted pupil, say during driving instruction or other individual tutorials. The participants have mutual respect (for the teacher's special knowledge and for the learner's personal invest- ment in the attempt to gain knowledge), may or may not like each other, but work together to reach a set of more or less concrete goals (passing the driving test, understanding the significance of death in the novels of Thomas Hardy). When these goals have been achieved, the two participants can go their separate ways because considerable independence between them has been maintained, in the sense that there are whole areas of their lives which are not involved in the relationship. So it is in cognitive-behavioural interviewing. Interviewers aim to intrude as little as possible into the lives of clients as possible, consistent with finding out what is needed to help them with their difficulties. Similarly, they offer personal information about themselves judiciously, in a manner consistent with appropriate self-disclosure to facilitate client change (Vandecreek & Angstadt, 1985). This is a key aspect of the fostering of client independence during a series of cognitive-behavioural interviews, and paves the way for uncomplicated ending interviews.

AIMS AND OBJECTIVES IN THE ENDING INTERVIEW

Aims

1 To close a series of interviews to the satisfaction of the client.
2 To arrange follow-up appropriately.
3 To cope with discharge of the unsuccessful client.
4 To decide about onward referral.

Objectives

1 To identify the optimum time to end a series of interviews
2 To describe to the client an appropriate rationale for ending and negotiate this process.

3 To negotiate with the client appropriate follow-up or onward referral arrangements.
4 To describe to the client how gains made may be maintained.

WHEN TO END A SERIES OF INTERVIEWS

Consideration of the timing of endings brings us back to the previous chapter, when we considered evaluation. In essence, therapeutic interventions should end *when the goals agreed between interviewer and interviewee have been achieved, or when they can agree that the achievement of these goals is unlikely to occur in the foreseeable future.* As with all elements of cognitive-behavioural interviewing, this is subject to negotiation between the two participants. Typically, then, ending occurs after some form of summative evaluation of the process and outcome of intervention, which itself forms a kind of final summary of what the work of the interviewer and interviewee has been about. It should be noted that this holds true for a range of interview types, not just for those interviews which contain active teaching or other intervention. The participants may, for example, have agreed to meet *only* for the purpose of assessment of a difficulty. Thus, when the nature of the difficulty has been established to the satisfaction of both, the goals of that series of interviews have been met in just the same way as goals of actively therapeutic interviews might be achieved, and the contract between interviewer and interviewee is at an end. There is no reason why assessment interviews should not be targeted in exactly the same quantitative way that we described in Chapter 5. Generally speaking, when intervention has been successful, there will be agreement between interviewer and interviewee that this is so, and that it is, therefore, appropriate to end their association. However, there may still be difficulties, particularly if the interviewer has not been effective in keeping the client orientated to the aims and process of the interviews. As we noted above, the ending process begins at the commencement of the first interview, through the process of client involvement and negotiation. As part of this process, the successful interviewer ensures that ending forms part of discussions with the client from an early stage in an intervention, and encourages the client to enter into continuing discussions which build towards discharge. The client may even be encouraged to tell the interviewer when ending is appropriate, perhaps after interim evaluations, so that finishing treatment comes as no surprise to the client, who, after successful intervention, may indeed welcome it and suggest it herself, as a response to 'next step' questions from the interviewer. In this sense, ending an intervention is no different from any other negotiation of a therapeutic step.

However, there is no doubt that some clients, however successful interactions with the interviewer have been, remain uncertain about their ability to maintain or increase the gains they have made during treatment. Once again, the suggestions regarding the negotiation of intervention with the client apply as much here as at other stages in the therapeutic relationship. If anything, the client has a stronger role to play in this part of intervention than in any other, as she prepares herself to take an even more active role in her care. To help with this, the sensitive interviewer makes particular use of attempts to facilitate the client in self-reassurance about the efficacy of intervention strategies she has learnt and prompts her to describe how she intends to continue to employ these strategies after the end of formal treatment, emphasizing the importance of self-rewards, setting of agendas and negotiating with herself about appropriate 'next steps' and fallback positions. In so doing, the interviewer aims to make explicit the rationale for ending intervention, as the end point in a process whereby the client becomes increasingly competent in organizing her owing coping resources. The nurse attempts to illustrate to the client that her role as nurse is now redundant in helping the client with her difficulties, since she herself now has sufficient knowledge or skill to fulfil that role.

Having established that interventions negotiated with the client have been effective, usually by a period of continuing monitoring during the later stages of the cycle of interviews, there is often no need for formal follow-ups of long duration at frequent or infrequent intervals. Where it is known that the client has a complaint which is likely to recur, such formal follow-ups are, indeed, required, but these do not necessarily involve the interviewer, who may have little or no responsibility for the formal medical care of the client. In both such instances, the requirement at discharge is again for negotiation between interviewer and interviewee as to their respective roles in specifying what will occur in the future. Naturally, some of these aspects will be quite routine, and governed by institutional convention. Here, the interviewer provides the client with precise information about such arrangements. Over and above these simpler institutional elements (letters to GPs, arrangement of adjunctive services such as transport to physiotherapy, outpatients appointment, home help), the aim of the interviewer is, wherever possible, to devolve as many practical tasks to the client as possible, in terms of arranging other appointments or contact arrangements. The interviewer only becomes involved with such arrangements as a facilitator, either advising the client on how to go about such arrangements or interceding where there has been evidence of administrative or other institutional difficulties. Once again, this is consistent with the notion of enabling the client to function assertively in taking responsibility for her health care. However, the successful interviewer recognizes that institutions can be difficult for outsiders, and responds sensitively to difficulties experienced by clients. Over and above this, the client simply needs accurate information about what will happen after ending: for example, contact by the interviewer with the referral agent, arrangements for re-referral if things go wrong in the future and how to maintain the gains made during intervention.

Where there still remains some uncertainty about long-term improvement, even though treatment has generally been successful, the interviewer may negotiate with the client that contact may be resumed without the need for a lengthy formal re-referral procedure, and many institutions have administrative conventions which allow this flexibility. It is, however, best to negotiate limits to this open access system with the client, since this is a way of conveying to her that continuing progress is thought by the interviewer to be likely. For example:

Inter:　So, although we've agreed that, in general, things are better and that we're going to stop meeting after today, there are still one or two areas which need some work. I'm going to suggest that you contact me again after two months if there's no further improvement, and we can talk again about how to proceed.

or, by contrast:

Inter:　So, things seem OK at present, and have been for the last few meetings. However, as we discussed, these problems can tend to come and go, so it's difficult to know for sure whether treatment is effective, or whether its just a random and temporary improvement. Of course, we both very much expect the improvement will be permanent, but just in case it proves not to be so, I'm going to offer you the opportunity to just phone me any time over the next six months, if things seem to be getting worse again, and we can meet again at fairly short notice and discuss what might be done. After that time, we can be fairly sure that the improvement will be for good, and I would say any further trouble would be very unlikely. If anything did crop up, you could get in touch with me through your GP in the normal way.

Returning to the issue of the need to maintain and consolidate gains after intervention has finished, the negotiation of how to go about this is similar to the negotiation of client interim goals at any stage during treatment, with three major differences. The client will then be *unable to seek further guidance* and feedback from the interviewer. This places an additional burden on both to ensure success-ful maintenance of intervention gains. As well as encouraging the self-maintenance tactics mentioned above, the interviewer will be careful, therefore, to ensure that the client has even more opportunity than usual to ensure she has understood what is required. The goals themselves will be different, in that they will often be *open-ended*, and so the client will need to be reminded of the need to continue to evaluate her success and to construct further goals independently of the interviewer. Lastly, the interviewer will have *no opportunity* either to *modify* her instructions to the client or to *reinforce* the client for appropriate performance, so that final reinforcements to her during the ending interview are of particular importance in maintaining compliance after intervention has ceased. The final interview offers a powerful opportunity for reinforcement of the client, since she is offered the ultimate assurance of the appropriateness of her performance – discharge. Such an opportunity should not be wasted or hurried, since the skilled interviewer will wish to minimize the likelihood of a reduction in adherence to the therapeutic interventions which have been painstakingly negotiated during the previous interviews, with consequent decrease in client well-being.

Unfortunately, not all our interventions with clients are successful, and in those cases where improvement is either modest or absent, particular care is needed in ending the interview cycle. It is not unreasonable for clients to feel disappointed or angry when told that there is no further help the nurse can currently give. Although this disappointment and anger should be acknowledged and handled by the interviewer in the same way as any other client emotions, it is particularly threatening, since it carries the implication with it of failure by the interviewer. This in turn may inhibit the interviewer's ability to deal with the client's response to discharge with sufficient sensitivity (Maguire, 1991). Additionally, despite the fact of the client's discomfort, it is often true that the interviewer really does have nothing more to offer, other than acknowledgement, and that the future may, as a result, be bleak for the client. As a result, there may be resistance to discharge, on the part of the interviewer as well as the client. The impulse to retain the client within the therapeutic relationship for 'just a little longer' should, however, be strongly resisted. In part, this desire stems from our need to be as helpful as possible to as many people as possible. Unfortunately, this need overlooks the reality that all manner of factors outside the control of our good intentions combine to make it impossible for us to help everyone we meet in interview situations, as they do in life more generally. For example, there may be elements of the client's personal circumstances which render it impossible, despite the best efforts of both herself and the interviewer, for her to put into practice those tactics which will cause improvement to her difficulties. Equally, the state of our knowledge, both as individuals and as a discipline may mean that we have inadequate experience or skill to guide her to such tactics even though these do, in fact, exist. Lastly, effective interventions for the client's difficulties may have yet to be developed.

These issues should be shared with the client, wherever possible in the context of attempting to offer some alternative to her, but if necessary, whilst admitting that no alternative is currently possible. Although both these circumstances represent a sad end, their frank discussion has the advantage of increasing the client's access to information, and, therefore, the likelihood of her having the best possible chance of reorganizing her life, whether through the seeking of some alternative intervention or the attempt to accommodate to those difficulties which currently remain insoluble.

Two particular elements of the discharge of unimproved clients require special mention. These are the issues of what constitutes an adequate trial of treatment, and what to do about onward referral of such clients. With regard to adequate and inadequate trials of treatment, this is a difficult, highly subjective matter, which is often again confused by our desire to help the client, and our consequent tendency to assume that unsuccessful interventions *would* be successful given a few more weeks, a shift of approach, and so on. The problem is compounded by the fact that these changes might well *truly* result in improvement for the client. Nevertheless, we cannot keep clients in treatment forever in the hope that this will turn out to be so. Thus, we need to develop personal criteria for deciding what constitutes an adequate trial of treatment for the unsuccessful client, so as to lessen the risk both of keeping them in treatment too long, and thus fostering additional dependency, or discharging them prematurely. As with successful ending, therefore, it can be seen that the discharge of the unsuccessful client also shares with other 'next steps' in treatment the need to find the most reinforcing step under the given circumstances. The following additional guide-lines in ensuring the trial of treatment has been adequate are suggested:

Enlist the client's help in understanding why treatment has not been successful.
Monitor progress during treatment sufficiently to ensure client understanding, client compliance, appropriateness of goals.
Renegotiate intervention tactics and goals when non-improvement becomes apparent.
Reassess the problem when non-improvement becomes apparent.
Be familiar with the success rate of a particular intervention, and use this to inform decisions about ending
Be familiar with the normative timescale for response to a particular intervention, and use this to inform decisions about ending.
Be flexible in the use of varying approaches to ensure client compliance, and examine the literature for *demonstrably effective* alternative approaches you have not tried.
By contrast, do not clutch at therapeutic straws.

Onward referral is often problematic for reasons which are similar to difficulties experienced with ending interventions with the unsuccessful client. Our doubts with regard to our self-worth may lead to our hesitating to refer a client on, whist our desire to be helpful may lead to our referring the client to another professional with only the vaguest idea of why we are so doing. Additionally, it is far easier to refer on than to say to a client: 'this is the end of the road'. Indeed, these two issues contribute to the tendency of clinicians to refer clients on and on and on in the hope that eventually there will be some 'expert' who will be able to help the person (Main, 1957). Unfortunately, there is often no basis for this hope, and onward referral only delays the moment when the client will have to come to terms with the fact that no hope is currently available, with the result that she is likely to be even further demoralized than by a frank admission of the true state of affairs. Even when the client actively seeks onward referral, in the absence of any potentially useful agency, the sensitive interviewer addresses this as a request for reassurance that 'everything will be all right', recognizes the ineffectiveness of this kind of reassurance, and responds accordingly by discussing the client's feelings about the issue and emphasizing her current strengths and coping abilities. It is inappropriate to offer hope where none is, in fact, on offer.

Equally, there are times when a different approach is highly appropriate, and in this case it is the duty of the nurse to discuss this with the client in such a way as to ensure that the most relevant referral is made. This will generally include the following aspects:

Agreement with the client as to the problems of the current intervention.
Agreement as to what remains to be done.
Discussion of the style of intervention the client would prefer (physical, medication, psychological, and so on).

Discussion of how much time and effort she can commit to the intervention proposed, including physical aspects (distance, travel arrangements).
Agreement of a timescale before referral should take place.
Agreement as to the role of the interviewer in facilitating the referral.
Agreement as to the amount of confidentiality required by the client in the making of the referral.
'Expert advice' from the interviewer about the appropriateness of potential alternative interventions.

ENDING THIS BOOK

Our discussion of ending a series of interviews brings us also about to the end of this book. Some of the issues addressed in this final chapter are as true for you as readers as they are for your clients. I am sure that I won't have addressed all of the questions and ideas you have about interviewing, and no doubt large areas remain where you are wondering where to go next, both practically and in terms of expanding your knowledge regarding the process of interviewing. It is with this in mind that the exercises associated with this chapter focus primarily upon your needs as an interviewer coming to the end of one phase in your search for excellence in interviewing. Like the completing client, you will need to devise strategies to monitor the continuing gains you intend to make as you carry on interviewing, to consolidate on those gains and to take appropriate action in the event that difficulties occur. Nor is it any mistake that I have concluded this book on the slightly negative note of discussion of the unsuccessful client. I am not predicting that your own interviews will likewise be unsuccessful: quite the reverse. Nevertheless, you will, most surely, have many clients whom you are able to help to only a slight degree, or are, perhaps, unable to help at all. Given the current state of our knowledge about human physical and mental processes, this is inevitable. What we can do, however, is to ensure that we deal with those clients with whom we are in contact to the best of our abilities, and ensure that those abilities are themselves as well-tuned as they can possibly be under the given circumstances. Hopefully, this book will have represented a step towards these goals.

CLINICAL EXAMPLE

Here, Jenny, a health visitor, concludes an ending interview with Gemma, a young mother who sought her advice regarding her son's 'temper tantrums', which have now resolved. They have already evaluated the interventions used.

Jenny: OK, so from what you tell me, it looks like things are going well with Andrew, and I wonder where we should go from here?

Gemma: Yes, well, I'm fairly happy with how things are.

Jenny: So, tell me, do you feel as if we should meet again?

Gemma: No, I don't think so, I feel as if I know enough now to know what to do if he starts up again.

Jenny: Yes, I think so, too. Can you just run through for me what you would do? (*Encouraging rehearsal, self-advising, checking contingency management tactics.*)

(*After a description from Gemma of the tactics she will use, Jenny proceeds to offer reinforcement.*)

Jenny: Yes, that's excellent, and I think it shows how hard you have worked at putting the things we spoke of into practice. Now, I want to just check how you're going to make sure that things *don't* start to get difficult again, and also if there are any things you plan on working on by yourself, to consolidate the gains. (*Checking how gains will be maintained and increased.*)

Gemma: I'll continue with the diary-keeping for a few more weeks, just to be certain, and make especially sure I don't respond if Andrew does lose his temper a little, so that I don't start to give him the attention for it. I'll also be really careful to give him plenty of praise for keeping his temper. As regards working on other things, I don't really think so. Sure, he's still naughty occasionally, but all children are.

Jenny: You feel that's pretty normal?

Gemma: Yes, I do.

Jenny: OK. That all sounds absolutely fine. How would you like to leave things as regards contact with myself? (*Preparing to negotiate follow-up.*)

Gemma: I was hoping just to be able to give you a ring, if things started to go wrong again.

Jenny: Yes, that sounds fine. The only thing I would suggest is that, if things do seem to be getting difficult again, you don't ring me straight away. You've done a good deal of the work during our time together, and have the knowledge you need to deal with any setbacks which might possibly crop up. (*Reinforcing client's own coping ability.*) Maybe we could agree that you'd try some of the tactics we spoke about again, for say a couple of weeks after you identified that things had become difficult to control, and then phoned if there was no improvement. (*Specifying a limit.*) I think it would just be a case of me offering a bit of 'fine tuning advice' to the skills you've already got. (*Final reinforcement.*)

Gemma: Yes, that sounds OK.

In the next example, Pete, a behaviour therapist, is in the unfortunate position of having to discharge a client, an agoraphobic man, with whom treatment has not been successful. The difficulty is compounded by the fact that behaviour therapy is the treatment of choice for this complaint, and that there is no reliable evidence that other treatments have anything to offer. Once again, evaluation has taken place, and several approaches have been negotiated and tried, all to no effect. There has been some difficulty on the part of the client, Dave, in complying with treatment instructions, because he found it difficult to accept the notion of decreasing anxiety following prolonged exposure.

Pete: Well, Dave, this is very difficult for me to say, but I feel, on the basis of what we have said in evaluating treatment so far, that there is nothing else we can do together to work on your difficulties.

Dave: Yes, I thought you would say so. I know I have found it difficult to do what we said. I wonder if there's anything else to be done?

Pete: It's unfortunate, but, at this stage, I don't think so. (*Resisting offering Dave further intervention.*) Although some little progress has been made, quite honestly, at the rate thing are going, I don't think coming here to see me adds anything to your own efforts, and we've already been though the need for more practice if any real improvement is going to occur, at least in the short term. We've met now on 15 occasions, and really things are little different. We've also tried several approaches, and, similarly, that has led to little change. (*Emphasizing the adequacy of the trial of treatment.*) I think, at this stage, we need to consider your options, and I myself feel you should have a break from formal therapy, so as to consider the future.

Dave: Is there some other form of treatment I could try?

Pete: Yes, there are a number of options. Unfortunately I have to tell you that there is much less evidence that these are effective than there is for the treatment you and I have been working with. Medication is of little use, and there is also no indication that traditional psychotherapy is helpful, so I wouldn't wish to refer you to either of those forms of intervention, unless you absolutely insisted. I must also say that I *am* a behaviour therapist, and so am naturally biased towards the sorts of treatment I offer, which as you know, are very much at odds with both drug treatment and psychoanalytic therapy. But at the same time I am giving you the best information that I know of. (*Resisting onward referral to ineffective therapies.*) At the same time, I am reluctant to refer you to another behaviour therapist. I know we have not been successful, but I do think we have done everything that can be done within the confines of behaviour therapy, and I'm not aware of anyone who has developed any new approaches within the behavioural field, so I wouldn't want to refer you on just for the sake of it, and just to disappoint you more. (*Frank admission of lack of success, but resistance of inappropriate re-referral to 'pass the buck'.*) I'm sure much of this is pretty depressing news, and I hope we can now talk about the impact it has on you. (*Acknowledging the effect of his words and inviting exploration of this.*)

(After a discussion of Dave's feelings about discharge, Pete continues:)

I am conscious that you may feel differently, however, and, once again, I would re-refer you if you absolutely insisted. Also, I should be prepared to see you again after some time has passed, and I should also like then to hear from you how things would be different, particularly with regard to the issue of frequent exposure that we mentioned earlier. (*Specifying future plans for a 'next step' with the client, specifying what went wrong in treatment and what, therefore, needs to be addressed before further intervention.*) I would suggest that you wait about six months, and then contact your GP to have him refer you again. (*Specifying the conditions by which re-referral will occur.*)

Pete then concludes by examining with Dave the possible tactics he can employ in dealing with his handicap alone, reinforces the need for continuing approach to the avoided situations and agrees practical arrangements such as contacting Dave's GP.

EXERCISES

1 Devise a checklist of the practical arrangements involved in discharging a client from your own clinical setting.

2 Use the reflective journal to assess your performance during a discharge interview. Pay particular attention to:

   client reinforcement;
   instructions on maintenance of gains;
   ensuring understanding of any practical arrangements.

3 Devise a programme of reading for yourself, using the suggestions given at the end of each chapter. Review your performance on this programme at the end of three months.

4 Identify a source of long-term support or supervision in interviewing from among your colleagues and agree a format for this support. As a starting point, you may wish to use the reflective strategies discussed in Chapter 3.

5 List potential difficulties you see in maintaining your current level of interviewing excellence and generate a series of tactics for addressing these difficulties.

6 Review this book and decide on its most serious shortcomings. Decide how you will work to make good this shortfall within the context of your own area of clinical practice.

7 Decide on a series of rewards for your continuing good practice (perhaps there is a particular book from the reading lists you would like to buy, or an important conference you would like to attend). Make these contingent on achieving the goals you set yourself for continuing excellence in interviewing

FURTHER READING

Davis, H. & Fallowfield, L. (1991) *Counselling and Education in Health Care.* Chichester. Wiley.

Appendix 1
Interview self-assessment form

Decide which aspects of the interview you want to concentrate on. Remember that it is hard to assess a whole interview at once, that not all issues on the form will apply to every interview, and that which elements you have covered depends on how much of the book you have read. Tick yes or no depending on whether you think a behaviour was performed by you appropriately or not.

Interviewer behaviour	Performed appropriately	
	YES	NO
Stated name and role	....	....
Established client's name	....	....
Stated timescale and agenda	....	....
Sought feedback about client's views on agenda	....	....
Explained any distractions	....	....
Made links with previous interviews/clinicians	....	....
Proceeded from general to specific	....	....
Used open questions	....	....
Used closed questions to get detail	....	....
Rewarded client information	....	....
Rewarded client coping	....	....
Used simple language	....	....
Negotiated with client	....	....
Offered aids to memory	....	....
Offered opportunities for modelling	....	....
Final reinforcement	....	....
Final negotiation and planning	....	....
Feedback from client	....	....

Appendix 2
Interviewing a client with chronic pain

Excerpts from a series of interviews are presented, in order to demonstrate the continuity of the cognitive-behavioural approach to interviewing through the various stages of the therapeutic process. Not *every* aspect of the each interview is presented, in the interests of space, and, as in the case material presented during each chapter, the client's remarks are abbreviated, since the main focus of the account is on interviewer behaviour.

BACKGROUND

The client, Barbara Jones, has been referred to the pain clinic by her GP. Ms Jones has experienced severe headaches for several years following a head injury sustained whilst working as a care assistant. The nurse, Hannah Irving, has spent several years specializing in the care of people with chronic pain, using a variety of different interventions.

INTERVIEW 1

Hannah opens the interview with introductory material and then proceeds with an examination of the client's difficulties. A rationale for treatment is presented. She closes by negotiating some interim work by the client and setting the scene for measurement of Barbara's difficulties during the next session.

Hannah: Hello. Barbara Jones?

Barbara: That's right.

Hannah: Hello, Mrs Jones. My name is Hannah Irving, and I'm one of the nurses here at the clinic. I've set aside an hour for our appointment, and, during that time, I hope to get as clear a picture of the issues that have brought you here today as I can. Before we start, though, I want to explain a bit about myself and what you can expect to happen during the interview. Is that OK? (*Name, role and agenda stated. Permission sought to continue.*)

Barbara: Yes, of course.

Hannah: Well, my job here at the clinic is to work with people who have had pain which has not gone away, for some time, despite medical treatments.

Barbara: That's me, worst luck!

Hannah: From the way you say that, it sounds as though it's been a very trying time for you. (*Reflection*). What I try and do is to work with people to help them find out what they themselves can do both to help cope with the pain and to lessen the amount of pain they get, without adding any new medicines. Quite how successful that is depends on a number of things, many of which are particular to every individual. That's why this interview is especially important, since it is over the next hour that I'll try, with your help, to get the best information possible regarding how the problem affects your life. (*Orientating the client, stressing the importance of the interview in order to increase likelihood of client attention and accurate information-giving.*) By the end of the conversation, you can expect that I will have made a decision, from my point of view, as to whether the treatments I offer can help. I will also explain these to you, give you the chance to ask questions, and ask you to say whether, so far as *you* are concerned, it is something you feel you want to go ahead with. If it turns out either that I don't feel I can help, or that you don't feel what I offer is for you, then I shall certainly discuss that issue with you, and we can talk about other options. Anyway, that's enough from me. I am now wondering whether this is the kind of thing you had in mind when you agreed to come here. If not, we can discuss that, too.

Even at this early stage, Hannah seeks to enlist the client's help, by describing likely outcomes and stressing the collaborative nature of treatment. She continues by using a statement (I am now wondering . . .) as a question to check the appropriateness of the agenda. After some general remarks by the client about her expectations, it is agreed that the interview can proceed.

Hannah: I have read your letter from your doctor, Dr Higgins, and I've also had the chance to look at your notes from Ancaster Hospital. (*Making links with previous consultations, and demonstrating relevant expertise through stressing that she has prepared.*) However, I think it is probably best at this stage for you to help me by telling me yourself what the main difficulties are at the moment. (*General, open question expressed as a statement.*)

Barbara: Well, it all started three years ago, when I was working in an old folks home. There was this old gentleman, and he was inclined to get a bit aggressive. Not violent, really, if you know what I mean, but, anyway, he took a swing at one of the other gentlemen. I don't know what it was about, but I grabbed his arm, and as a result, I fell over and banged my head on the edge of a table. There was blood everywhere ... (*Barbara continues in this vein for some time.*)

Hannah: OK, so it began about three years ago and you hit you head very hard (*summarizes*), but let me, just to be clear, bring you right up to the present, so I can get a picture of the problems now. (*Redirects the client so as to orient both to the original question.*)

Barbara: Oh, sorry.

Hannah: Not at all, I agree that it's very important to talk about how it started, and we'll certainly do that later. (*Stresses that client concerns will be examined.*)

Barbara: Well, at the moment, it's the headaches that are the worst problem, although the flashing lights and the dizziness seem to come and go, too.

Hannah: OK. Let's look at the headaches, first, then, since that's what you describe as the worst difficulty. Can you describe what they feel like? (*Specific, open question.*)

Barbara: It's as though there's a tight band round your head, and it goes on being tightened as time goes on. It's mainly here (indicates back of head), but sometimes very bad here (indicates right side of head).

Hannah: So, a band round the head, mainly feels painful at the back, but sometimes here (indicates side of head)? (*Paraphrasing.*) So that I can get an idea of how severe it is, can you tell me what you do when you get an episode? (*Orientating the client, exploring behaviour and impact on her life.*)

Barbara: Most of the time, I'd take some medication immediately. I've found that if I leave it, it takes longer to work. Now, I tend to go and lie on the bed, and draw the curtains.

Hannah: I see, thank you. (*Reinforcing information-giving by Barbara.*) Still looking at what you do, suppose you're out and you feel an episode occurring?

Barbara: If that happens I feel I have to get home as soon as possible, but I tend not to go out much now. Certainly not on my own, because it can be so awful if I get pain then.

Hannah: Yes. I think I can see how that must be very distressing ... Can I ask roughly how often you're getting the headaches now? (*Specifier.*)

Barbara: Certainly every day. Sometimes more.

Hannah: And for roughly how long on each occasion? (*Specifier.*)

Barbara: It depends, it can go on for hours.

Hannah: That must be very difficult. Are there any thoughts that run through your mind while this is going on? (*Eliciting cognitions associated with the problem episodes.*)

Barbara: Mainly, I just wish it will end. Sometimes I think it never will, especially if it's a bad attack. Sometimes I'm scared that something is happening to me.

Hannah: Can you tell a bit more about that? (*Seeking clarification.*)

Barbara: As though all this pain must mean I'm being harmed. You know, that it's damaging me. As though I'm going to have a stroke.

Hannah: That sounds so frightening. I think particularly when the pain is actually there. (*Reflection.*)

Barbara: Yes. I try and distract myself, think about other things, but the pain always breaks through.

Hannah: Is that a general rule, that the pain stops you concentrating? (*Closed question eliciting problem severity.*)

Barbara: Yes.

> *At this point, Hannah has concentrated primarily on the client's experience when a painful episode is occurring. She asks further questions and discovers that, by and large, the pain is worse when Barbara is by herself, and worse in the evening. If her husband is present, he generally comforts her, and takes over anything Barbara might be doing, something which she hates. Hannah summarizes before going on to ask about the antecedents and consequences of the painful episodes.*

Hannah: Can you tell me something about what happens just before a headache starts? (*Open question.*)

Barbara: Well, I get a slight feeling of tightness round the head, and I often feel very tense then.

Hannah: Tense in what way? (*Seeking clarification and helping the client to clarify.*)

Barbara: Well, in the body, sort of. All my muscles seem very tight. Not just in the head, but almost all over.

Hannah: It sounds as if you're anticipating what's going to happen. (*Confronting.*)

Barbara: Very much so. You get so used to the signs. The tightness and the flashing lights. It's almost like expecting it to happen.

Hannah: So, before an episode, you'd experience the flashing lights and the tightness. Also some muscle tension. (*Recapping.*) Any other physical sensations?

Barbara: Erm. No, that's it.

Hannah: Earlier, we mentioned the thoughts you have when a headache occurs. Can I ask you once again about thoughts that run through your mind, but this time before an episode. (*Hannah keeps the client orientated by referring to an earlier part of the interview and linking it to the present. Rather than pursuing her examination of the three systems in a mechanical way, she has followed the client's own discourse. In response to the general question beginning this section, Barbara replied by talking about physical symptoms, which Hannah pursued. She is then free to move, in a logical way, to examine behaviour and cognition antecedent to the problematic episodes. The interview proceeds by examining consequences in a similar, client-led way. Following this, Hannah feels she has a clear picture of Barbara's difficulties. She has also ensured that Barbara has had the relevant tests to exclude any continuing organic difficulties. In the excerpt that follows, she offers Barbara a summary of the interview and invites questions and comments, before offering a rationale for the interventions which she will suggest.*)

Hannah: So, let me first of all thank you again for giving me such helpful information. (*Reinforcement.*) I know it is often difficult to talk about things which cause such distress. At this point, I want to try and summarize the things we've touched on, so as to see I've got it right from your point of view. At the moment, you get severe headaches at the back and sometimes side of the head. The pain happens at least every day, and can go on for hours at a time, though the average length of time is about one and a half hours. When you get pain, it is generally so severe that you have to take medication and lie down in a dark room, and the pain makes you very afraid. At other times, you will often avoid doing things, in case you get an attack, and we ran through a list of some of those things. They include reading, watching television, going far from home, driving, dancing, swimming, jogging, having sex with your husband, and playing with your little boy. All of which you would rather do. To be fair, you say you are mainly worried that these activities will spark off an attack, but haven't noticed any specific connection. Finally, I should mention that we spoke about some of the physical sensations you had, and also talked about your thoughts and fears at these times in some detail. Well, I seem to have said a lot, but now it's over to you, and I'm really keen to hear whether you think I've got a reasonable idea of your difficulties. Please add anything you want to. Afterwards, I'll be going on to discuss with you what we might do. (*Emphasizing collaboration.*)

Barbara: No, what you say seems just about right. But I wonder what can be done. It's been going on for so long.

Hannah: Yes, I'm sure it must seem like that. If it's OK, I'd like to say a bit about how we might go on?

Barbara: (Nods).

Hannah: Well, to begin with, we've agreed that all the tests you've had have failed to come up with anything to account for why you still have headaches so long after the initial injury. I must say straightaway that that doesn't mean your pain isn't real. Unfortunately, it also doesn't mean *absolutely* that there's nothing wrong. As you know, medical tests are not infallible, and I know one of your great fears is that something dangerous is going on that you're not aware of. I can only say that, as far as the state of our knowledge is concerned at present, that is extremely unlikely, particularly given that your symptoms have not changed over the years. It seems most likely that the damage you received initially, although still causing pain, is not going to increase. And I think that is the message you've had from your consultant in the past. (*Avoiding blanket reassurance of the client, in favour of a detailed description of the likely current situation.*)

This leaves us with the problem of what to do about the pain you now experience. I think there are a number of tactics we could try, and I'll outline them in a minute. First, I should say two things: the techniques I have used benefit the majority of people whom I see. Nowhere near all of these people go away free of pain, but about two thirds report a major reduction in levels of pain, whilst a further 20 per cent report that they are able to live a more normal, productive life, in spite of pain. (*Prediction of likelihood of success.*) So you can see only about 10–15 per cent get no benefit at all. Also, there is nothing dangerous to the treatment I offer, and it doesn't mean you have to stop the physiotherapy. That can go on alongside of what we do together.

The intervention, then. Firstly, it's important, I think, to note that you've already made a lot of attempts to help yourself with these difficulties; for instance, the relaxation exercises, and that you still manage to do a great many things, in spite of the difficulties. (*Reinforcing coping attempts.*) We will build on these efforts during treatment. It is now fairly well known that pain, tension and fearful thoughts are closely linked, and, under some circumstances, combine to reinforce each other – the more pain, the more tension, the more fearful thoughts, the more tension, the more pain, and so on. Often, this is associated with avoiding certain behaviours, such as you have described. This in turn leads to low mood, and the pain can come to dominate the whole life, because of its consequences and effects on the life. (*Description of her view of the problem.*) Treatment aims to decrease pain through decreasing tension and fear and increasing activity levels so as to help with mood and general levels of well-being. So as to do these things, we will negotiate together specific interventions. I suggest we'll try a different form of relaxation exercise, which you'll learn and practise here, with my assistance. We'll also start to schedule a series of activities of increasing difficulty, which you yourself would like to do, but have been avoiding because of the pain. Doing these things again is beneficial in itself because it leads to increased effectiveness and self-esteem in your life, providing you are successful. Part of my job is to help you schedule the activities in such a way as to *maximize* your chances of success, so that you don't get demoralized by the size of the task. The other advantage of reintroducing activities is that you test out for yourself whether the things you fear will actually occur, and, by facing the fears themselves, allow them to diminish – just like going into a frightening interview and making yourself remain till the end. Finally, we'll work directly to alter the things you say to yourself at times of pain, since frightening thoughts tend to increase painful experience. (*General description of proposed interventions.*) For instance, we may agree that you start jogging again – just for a few minutes a day to begin with, while keeping a diary to record whether this has any effect on pain frequency and levels. We'll also negotiate a gradual introduction of activities to be done even when pain *is* happening, to demonstrate to yourself just how much you are capable of, even at the worst of times. (*Specific examples of client behaviour.*) I will be involved in guiding you with this. We'll meet here on a weekly basis, for about ten weeks, and work out and negotiate the schedules for the work your going to be doing, as well as practising relaxation and challenging the frightening thoughts. (*Description of nurse activities, mention of negotiation.*)

After some questions from Barbara and clarification from Hannah, Barbara agrees to give treatment a try. In what follows, the session closes with some interim goal-setting and an orientation of the client to the areas to be covered at the next meeting. Finally, Hannah attends to the principles of effective closure discussed in Chapter 5:

Hannah: At this point, I hope we can negotiate a number of things for you to do between now and next time. I think these will be important in helping us gain more precise information about the problem, and will also set the scene for some of what we do next time, when I'll come on to talk about measurement of your progress. The first thing I want to suggest is keeping a diary of the pain episodes. (Shows diary form.) This will help clarify how far your life is affected, and I hope you'll be able to fill it in, as far as possible, when the painful episodes are actually occurring. Have a look at it and see what you think. Remember we can always modify things which you think are too difficult or too time-consuming.

Barbara: No, that's fine.

Hannah: Great! (*Reinforcement*.) The other thing I was hoping might happen is if you would be able to select one thing you avoid at the moment and have a try at doing it. The idea here is to prove to yourself that there are still things your are able to do, so it's important to pick something that you've a reasonable chance of success with. What do you think?

Barbara: Well, how about reading? I'd really like to be able to do that again, it would make such a big difference.

Hannah: I'm sure so. The only thing I'm thinking is that you might want to just go for short articles to start with. It could be very frustrating to start on something long and find you can't finish it, either because your concentration is poor, or because a headache starts up. I'm not predicting that *will* happen, but I know from my own experience how upsetting it can be to start something you can't finish. (*Self disclosure*.)

Barbara: Yes, I can see that. I've got a book of short stories. How about that?

Hannah: Perfect. Can we agree that you'll do that every day?

Barbara: (Nods)

Hannah: Good. Now, next time, when we meet, I hope to go into the issue of measuring your difficulties with you, so we'll have something to compare your eventual successes with. This will also help us to modify and rearrange the things we do together if we come across any snags in treatment. You will have the major role in setting these treatment goals, and I'll bring along a number of forms I use to help you with this. For the moment though, can I just check whether there are any things you want to ask me about before we close today's session and arrange to meet again? (*Final questions*.)

Barbara: No, I think it's OK.

Hannah: Good. Just to be certain I've explained things properly, though, can you just tell me what you're going to be doing over the next week? (*Seeking feedback on understanding*.)

Barbara: Well, I've to keep a diary of when and where I get pain. Also, I'm going to try starting to read again. Should I make a note of how I get on with that, too.

Hannah: Yes, that would be great. I should have thought to mention that. Thanks. (*Pauses.*) At this point, I think we're about finished for today. We've talked a lot about your difficulties and what might be done, and also agreed on how we'll go forward. I want to thank you once again for giving me such good information, and indeed for agreeing to work with me. I recognize that it is often very difficult to deal with issues which have been causing so much difficulty, and I think it's really good that you've been able to. (*Final summary and reinforcement of information-giving and coping commitment.*) Before we make practical arrangements, let me ask you whether this interview has met your expectations? (*Seeking final feedback on agenda.*)

Barbara: Well, different from what I thought. Better, in a way, actually. I'm glad that I can get to have my own say in what I'm expected to do.

Hannah: Thank you. Let's now go out into the secretary's office and make arrangements for the next appointment.

INTERVIEW 2

After initial greetings, Hannah reviews Barbara's performance of the tasks negotiated last week, then continues with goal-setting and measurement. Some interim targets are agreed, and Hannah and Barbara talk through tactics for meeting these targets.

Hannah: Last week, I talked about the notion of target-setting, and this week, I hope we'll go on to look at that in some detail. But first, tell me how you got on with the things we agreed last week.

Barbara: Better than I expected, actually! (*Hannah nods reinforcement.*) I read for 20 minutes every day, and only started a headache towards the end of one of the episodes.

Hannah: Excellent. What did you do when that happened? (*Seeking specificity.*)

Barbara: I carried on till the end of the 20 minutes.

Hannah: That's great. Can we have a look at the diary?

Hannah and Barbara discuss the diary at some length.

Hannah: Now to move on to goal-setting. Here, we're looking for some things which you would like to be able to do, but that you can't do at the moment, because of the way pain affects you. We've already agreed that it's pain that stops you doing many important things in your life, and later on I'm going to ask you for a direct measure of the severity of pain for you in general, and how far it interferes with you. At present, thought, I'm looking for a number of precise targets you can work towards, since we agreed that, if you could do them, this would, in itself, indicate your pain had gone down. In this way, we'll have different measures of pain in different contexts, as well as your general feeling. Can you think of something now which is important to you, and would show us a distinct improvement if it was achieved? (*Goal should be desired by client and express change.*)

Barbara: Well, of course, there's sex. That's a huge issue for my husband.

Hannah: Sure, I can appreciate that. How big an issue for you, though? (*Emphasizes client's ownership of goals.*)

Barbara: Yes, absolutely.

Hannah: OK, can we specify this a bit. How often would you want to have sex, if it wasn't for the pain? (*Eliciting frequency.*)

Barbara: (Chuckles) To be honest, anything at all would be good! No, I suppose twice a week. That's about how often we used to before.

Hannah: And what do you think would be a reasonable time to spend. I ask this because, there would be a tendency to cut it short if there was worry that a headache might happen, is that right? (*Seeking to specify duration and seeking feedback on inference.*)

Barbara: Well, I suppose we'd go up to the bedroom and spend about an hour there, fooling around. Not necessarily having sex the whole time, you understand.

Hannah: Sure. I've been noting what you said. See how this sounds: To have sex with my husband (*target behaviour*), twice a week (*frequency*), for an hour on each occasion (*duration*), in our bedroom (*setting*), continuing even if I fear I might start a headache (*criteria*).

Barbara: OK, but . . . surely there's no point in having sex if I've got pain?

Hannah: No, certainly not. It's the issue of *fear* of pain we're talking about here. Other exercises we're going to do will also help with the levels of pain. See how the target is supposed to be rated (*shows Figure 5.2*). *It does say: "without difficulty", and, for our purposes, that means that to achieve that target there should be no pain at the time, or at least, in the early stages of treatment, minimal discomfort.*

Barbara: OK, I've got that.

Hannah: Great. Now, here, I want you to rate how far you've got with that target, even before we start. This will give us an idea of how things are now and what we're to compare your improvement with. What you do is put a mark on the line to say how far you have achieved the target so far. So right down here at the zero end is no success at all yet, and 100 per cent means the target is totally achieved. Where are you on that line?

Barbara: Well, nought, I suppose. (Marks line)

Hannah: Yes, I know that seems distressing, but remember we are at the beginning of our work together. In one way, the fact that you score low is helpful. It means we've selected a target which, if you reach it, will indicate a major success. It's something to work towards for the end of treatment, not for today or next week.

Barbara: Thank you.

Hannah: Thank you. That's helpful. Can we now move on and set a target about a different area of your life that's affected.

Barbara: How about driving?

Hannah: Yes, that's a big one. If that was successful, that would make a big difference to you. Let's follow the same system as before. How often would you want to drive? (*Frequency.*)

Barbara: At the moment, I don't need to very often, but that's because my husband has taken over so much. In an ideal world, every day.

Hannah: Excellent, let's say daily, then – for the end of treatment, remember. And for how long on each occasion? (*Duration.*)

Barbara: (Smiles, getting the idea) Up to half and hour, by myself (*Criteria.*), and just in local areas (*Setting.*)

Hannah: (Laughs) Yes, that seems to cover about every aspect! Just bear with me while I get this down. (Writes) Have a look at the form and make your mark on the line.

Hannah: Now because, as we noticed last time, many areas of your life are affected, so we can't target every aspect, but it is important to try and get some more general coverage, so let's go on to select some other targets from different areas.

Hannah and Barbara negotiate several further targets, and Hannah stresses repeatedly that these are targets for the end of treatment. They then turn to the negotiation of interim goals for Barbara to attempt between this session and the next. One of these relates to the issue of car driving.

Hannah: What do you think would be a reasonable first step towards starting driving again?

Barbara: How about a short trip out once this week?

Hannah: Hmm. I think the idea of short trips is a good one (*Differential reinforcement.*), but I'm worried about the frequency. This would hardly give you any opportunity to get used to the apprehension you have.

Barbara: Well, I suppose I could manage twice.

Hannah: Brilliant. I think that would be very good, given the other things you're going to be working on as well. And we agree that you only start the drive if there is no pain present?

Barbara: Yes.

Hannah: Now take me through exactly what you're going to do the first time you go out in the car. (*Question phrased as statement. Talk-through.*)

Barbara: Well, I'll decide on a destination, and a maximum time to stay out. I'll drive slowly to begin with, until I get used to it, and stay in familiar territory.

Hannah: Yes, that seems right. If you get pain?

Barbara: Drive slowly home. Don't rush to get back to safety.

Hannah: Excellent. Tell me how you think you will feel if you manage this task? (*Encouraging automodelling.*)

Barbara: Very good indeed. I'll have done something I haven't managed for ages.

Hannah: Great. How will you reward yourself for that? (*Encouraging self-reinforcement.*)

The usual practical planning and seeking of feedback now take place.

INTERVIEW 3

Following review of the past week's events, Hannah and Barbara discuss specific difficulties in carrying out the agreed tasks. Modifications are suggested.

Hannah: Today, I thought we could start by having a look at how you've got on this week. Then I'd go through the relaxation exercises with you. Finally, we can plan what happens between now and next time. How does that sound?

Barbara: Fine.

Hannah: Good. Can you start us off, then, by saying a bit about how you got on with the things we agreed you'd be doing last week?

Barbara: Yes. On the whole it's gone quite well. I've got the diary here. (Passes diary) As you can see, I filled it in each day. It's interesting, because there seems to have been a bit less pain this week than usual.

Hannah: Yes, that's not unusual. It's strange, but many people report this. It's almost as though examining the experience of pain helps us get control over it. Anyway, it's certainly good that there's been a bit of a let-up this week. Thanks for keeping such precise information. Let's look at some of the week's goals. Which do you want to start with.

Barbara: The driving?

Hannah: OK.

Barbara: Well, I didn't find it too difficult, the first time. I had no pain, and although I was worried that I might have an attack, I managed to stay out the whole time. But . . . I went out again yesterday and started with a bad head almost as soon as I got in the car.

Hannah: That's bad news. Tell me what you did then.

Barbara: I just drove round the block, then I felt so bad that I had to come home, and I got straight up on the bed.

Hannah: OK. That sounds like it must have been quite a bad episode. What sort of thoughts ran through your head at the time?

Hannah now deals with the problematic episode during homework just like any other example of the client's difficulties, investigating the ABCs in search of specific maintaining factors which have contributed to difficulty. It turns out that Barbara had been experiencing a small amount of discomfort earlier in the morning, just prior to going out in the car, but had decided to 'tough it out', getting very tense as she got out of the door and into the car. She reports feeling the muscular tension increasing as she continued to drive, with resulting sharp increase in pain.

Hannah: Well, first of all, let me say I think it's very important that you're so involved with the treatment targets we set, and had a go even when you were feeling pretty poorly. (*Differentially reinforcing coping attitudes.*) The problem is that, on this occasion, you were, I think, trying a bit too hard for this stage in your attempts. How would you rectify that next time?

Barbara: You mean, not go out? Surely that's just like what I've been doing before?

Hannah: Yes, except that you don't stay in indefinitely. You wait until the pain has passed, then immediately go out at that point. You capitalize on the times at which you can cope to begin with, to stress that there are still possibilities of success for you in reaching this target. Later on, you could try going out when there is a greater risk of an episode occurring. How does that sound?

Barbara: That makes sense.

Hannah: So this week, then, how are you going to go about it?

Barbara: Could I add another trip out?

Hannah: Yes, that sounds good, but what about the tactics you're going to use?

Barbara: How do you mean?

Hannah: Sorry. Tell me about *when* you're going to try driving.

Barbara: At times when there's no pain.

Hannah: Good. And, if there is a hint of pain when you're about to go out?

Barbara: I'll wait until it passes, and then go out immediately.

Hannah: Excellent. I think it's particularly useful, then, that we're going to go on today to look at relaxation as a coping tactic. That'll be something you can use during your practice. But first let's examine the other targets we set.

The interview then goes on to examine these targets and teach the relaxation exercises, before negotiating further tasks for Barbara to perform between sessions.

INTERVIEW 5

An interim review of progress towards treatment goals is conducted. One goal is renegotiated.

Hannah: Well, I think we agreed last week that this session would be a review. We've been working together for about seven weeks, now, since we first met to assess your difficulties. I hope we should be able to see from your feedback whether we're on the right track now. You remember we filled in these forms together?

Barbara: Yes.

Hannah: Well, I'd like to start off today's session by looking at them again. I'm going to ask you to rate them in exactly the same fashion you did during our second session. Afterwards, I hope we'll talk at more length about how things have gone. (*Orientating the client, using explicit categorization, attempting to avoid bias in the ratings.*)

Hannah and Barbara now rate several of her pre-treatment targets, including:

Hannah: Now let's look again at the target regarding driving. You stated that you wanted to be able to drive each day, for up to half an hour, just driving locally. Can I ask you to make a mark on the line again, indicating how far you've now got towards achieving that goal?

Barbara: (Marks line)

Hannah: Thank you, that's excellent.

Barbara: Can I just say that I'd like to alter that target a bit?

Hannah: Certainly, but can we keep with the ratings for the present, so that we can keep a focus on it. I promise we'll talk about amending this target afterward. Is that OK? (*Avoiding bias by introduction of material which may be expected to affect the client's scores.*)

Barbara: Sure.

> *Barbara and Hannah now rate the rest of their targets. Hannah compares Barbara's current scores with her previous ones, as in the example below.*

Hannah: So, on the issue of driving, you were way out here at the zero end of the scale (shows scale), but this is improved to about half way (shows mid-treatment rating) – in fact, 52 per cent, if I measure it. To me that seems quite excellent, but you did say you wanted to talk about this particular target, so I've left it till last, so that we can spend a bit of time talking about it. What's the issue here for you?

Barbara: Well, I was thinking that, in fact, I don't need to go out quite every day, on the one hand, but, on the other, I'd like to be able to go further afield, though not on a regular basis.

Hannah: Thank you, I see the difficulty. The target we've got doesn't now seem as realistic. Can I check out how often you now think would be reasonable in a week?

Barbara: Perhaps five times?

Hannah: OK. And the longer journeys. How long would they be?

Barbara: Could be a couple of hundred miles, but only two or three times a month. You see, if I can get back to work, I might well have to do a little bit of travelling.

Hannah: Yes, I do see, and I also think it's pretty exciting that you can start to think about going back to work, *and* can talk in terms of a couple of hundred miles being just a *bit* of driving. That's excellent! (*Reinforcing coping attitudes.*) I have a suggestion. Let's set a further target to do with long journeys, and rate that separately. With regard to the frequency thing – how about rating it both ways, in future – for seven, and five times a week. Just to see if there's in fact a difference in how you would rate those two frequencies. It seems to me, if you can do something like this five times a week easily, another two is neither here nor there. (*Encouraging measurement tactics which avoid bias.*)

Barbara: Yes, that seems OK.

> *The interview continues.*

INTERVIEW 10

Barbara and Hannah have agreed that this will be the last session of formal treatment. By the time we join the interview, they have completed formal measurement, and are now discussing how the gains she has made have helped Barbara. They continue by agreeing plans for follow-up. Hannah elicits from Barbara her plans in terms of consolidating treatment gains during the posttreatment period.

Hannah: So if I were to summarize what you've written on the forms, there is still quite a bit there in the way of headaches, but they aren't daily any more. (*Question phrased as statement.*)

Barbara: Yes, about three a week.

Hannah: But what seems more important is both the duration and severity.

Barbara: Certainly they don't last for anything like as long, and I find the relaxation exercises usually help to get rid of them.

Hannah: Excellent, and in terms of severity?

Barbara: Pretty much what I put on the form really. No more than about half as bad, often milder than that.

Hannah: That's excellent. At this point, I want to stress the importance of what you are doing, too. From what you say, it seems that you're tackling most things now. There's the driving, of course, and you're also going out much more frequently, and then there's the TV.

Barbara: Yes, and reading, too. I find I can really concentrate. This will be important when I get back to work. There is still the business of sex, though.

Hannah: That's right, and you identified that as one of the first targets that we set together. To be fair, though, some improvement has been made in that area?

Barbara: Yes, that's right, James and I are making love again now, but we've only tried it once or twice, and it's all a little strained.

Hannah: How does that feel for you?

Barbara: Normal, in a sense, I guess. I mean, I don't think it has much to do with the problem of pain. Although, if it gets a bit strenuous, I do worry a little that it might spark off an episode.

Hannah: Thank you, that's helpful. I think, at this stage, that's a realistic fear. Can you suggest how you can go about tackling it.

Barbara: Well, I thought James and I might agree only to use certain positions, to begin with, and to go at it very gently. Just till I've got used to all the activity again!

Hannah: That sounds fine, but will you also agree to set limits on this in terms of time?

Barbara: How do you mean?

Hannah: Well, at the moment, I feel very much that it's OK to be apprehensive, but I also guess you wouldn't want that to go on for too long. I wonder how long seems reasonable to you?

Barbara: A couple of months.

Hannah: Yes, that seems right. After that, what might you do?

Barbara: Could I be referred here again?

Hannah: Sure. I think it will be OK just to phone up again for, let's say the next three months. After that, I'd ask that you go through your GP again, just since it seems reasonable that if things go on OK for that length of time they're likely, in my experience, to stay OK. How does that sound?

Barbara: Fine. I feel quite confident, in a way.

Hannah: Good. Can we just, now, use one of your successful targets as a means both of looking at how you can increase your gains on the longer term goals where some work still needs to be done, and as an example of what to do if there is any time when your difficulties start to increase again? Let's use the reading as an example. What will you do if you feel that it's starting to spark off headaches again?

Barbara: First of all, I'll leave everything the same for a while to be sure it isn't just a chance thing.

Hannah: Excellent.

Barbara: If things don't improve, I might try a bit of diary keeping, just to try and identify if anything else is changing.

Hannah: That sounds good, but I would suggest that you already start reintroducing the coping tactics we have used in the past, at this point, just to be on the safe side. Does that seem reasonable?

Barbara: Yes, that seems fine.

Hannah: Great. Let's have a look at the issue of long journeys. Any ideas about how to approach these?

Barbara: Well, just the same as the shorter ones, in a way. I thought I'd start by going as far as Watford.

Hannah: Hmm, yes. I think generally you're right. The general approach is the same. But Watford, I think, is a bit too near. You can more or less do that now. Given the success you've had so far, could we agree to pick something a bit further afield?

Barbara: (Laughs) Yes, OK.

Barbara and Hannah continue in this way for some minutes, identifying tactics to help Barbara consolidate the gains she has made. Both are aware that success has not been complete, but Barbara feels that pain has reduced, that she is able to cope more adequately with what pain remains, and that there is every likelihood of continuing improvement. Most importantly, she is left with the impression that both her past successes and her likely further improvements are the product of her own efforts.

References

Anderson, J.R. & Bower, G.H. (1973) *Human Associative Memory*. Washington, DC. Winston.

Argyle, M. (1969) *Social Interaction*. London. Tavistock.

Argyle, M. (1988) *Bodily Communication*. London. Routledge.

Ausubel, D.A, Novak, J.D. & Hanesian, H. (1978) *Educational Psychology: A Cognitive View*. New York. Holt, Rinehart & Winston.

Azrin, N.H. & Nunn, R.G. (1973) Habit reversal: a method of eliminating nervous habits and tics. *Behaviour Research & Therapy* 11, 619–928.

Baddeley, A. (1983) *Your Memory: A User's Guide*. Harmondsworth. Penguin.

Bailey, R. (1985) *Coping and Stress in Caring*. Oxford. Blackwell.

Bandura, A. (1977a) *Social Learning Theory*. Englewood Cliffs, NJ. Prentice Hall.

Bandura, A. (1977b) Self-efficacy: towards a unifying theory of behavioral change. *Psychological Review* 84, 191–215.

Barker, P.J. (1982) *Behaviour Therapy Nursing*. London. Croom Helm.

Beck, A.T. (1976) *Cognitive Therapy and the Emotional Disorders*. New York. International Universities Press.

Bille, D.A. (1981) *Practical Approaches to Patient Teaching*. Boston. Little, Brown & Co.

Birch, J. (1979) The anxious learners. *Nursing Mirror* (February 8), 17–24.

Brammer, L.M. (1988) *The Helping Relationship. Process and Skills*. Englewood Cliffs, NJ. Prentice Hall.

Brammer, L.M, Shostrom, E. & Abrego, P. (1988) *Therapeutic Psychology: Fundamentals of Counseling and Psychotherapy*. Englewood Cliffs, NJ. Prentice Hall.

Brewin, C. (1988) *Cognitive Foundations of Clinical Psychology*. Hove. Lawrence Erlbaum Associates.

Burnard, P. & Morrison, P. (1991) *Caring and Communicating: The Interpersonal Relationship in Nursing*. Basingstoke. Macmillan Education.

Chomsky, N. (1959) Review of Skinner's *Verbal Behavior*. *Language* 35, 26–58.

Clarke, M. (1987) Review article. *International Journal of Nursing Studies* 24, 2, 169–72.

Coid, J. (1991) Interviewing the aggressive patient. *In* R.Corney (ed.) *Developing Communication and Counselling Skills in Medicine*. London. Routledge.

Collins, A.M. & Quillian, M.R. (1972) Experiments in semantic memory and language comprehension. *In* L.W.Gregg (ed.) *Cognition in Learning and Memory*. New York. Wiley.

Coolican, H. (1990) *Research Methods and Statistics in Psychology*. London. Hodder & Stoughton.

Crow, J. (1979) Assessment. *In* C.R. Kratz (ed.) *The Nursing Process*. London. Bailliere Tindall.

Davis, H. & Fallowfield, L. (1991) *Counselling and Education in Health Care*. Chichester. Wiley.

Dewing, J. (1990) Reflective practice. *Senior Nurse* 10 (10) 26–8.

Dillon, J.T. (1990) *The Practice of Questioning.* London. Routledge.

Dryden, W. (1991) *A Dialogue with Arnold Lazarus: 'It Depends'.* Milton Keynes. Open University Press.

Dryden, W. & Ellis, A. (1986) Rational-emotive therapy. *In* W. Dryden & W.L. Golden (eds) *Cognitive-behavioural Approaches to Psychotherapy.* London. Harper & Row.

Dryden, W. & Golden, W.L. (eds) (1986) *Cognitive-behavioural Approaches to Psychotherapy.* London. Harper & Row.

Egan, G. (1990) *The Skilled Helper: A Systematic Approach to Effective Helping.* Pacific Grove, California. Brooks/Cole.

Ekman, P. & Friesen, V.W. (1971) Constants across cultures in the face and emotion. *Journal of Personality and Social Psychology* 17, 124–9.

Ellis, A. (1962) *Reason and Emotion in Psychotherapy.* New York. Lyle Stuart.

Ellis, A. (1983) How to deal with your most difficult client: You. *Journal of Rational-Emotive Therapy* 1 (1), 3–8.

ENB (English National Board for Nursing Midwifery and Health Visiting) (1989) *Managing Change in Nursing Education. Pack Two: Workshop Materials for Action.* London. ENB.

Fairburn, C.G. & Cooper, P.J. (1989) Eating disorders. *In* K. Hawton, P.M. Salkovskis, J. Kirk, & D.M. Clark, (eds) *Cognitive-Behaviour Therapy for Psychiatric Problems. A Practical Guide.* Oxford. Oxford University Press.

Farrell, G.A. & Gray, C. (1992) *Aggression: A Nurses' Guide to Therapeutic Management.* London. Scutari.

Fraser, M. (1990) *Using Conceptual Nursing in Practice. A Research-based Approach.* London. Harper & Row.

Ghosh, A., Marks, I.M. & Carr, A.C. (1988) Therapist contact and outcome of self-exposure treatment for phobias. *British Journal of Psychiatry* 152, 234–8.

Goldberg, D.P., Hobson, R.F., Maguire, G.P., Margison, F.R., O'Dowd, T., Osborn, M. and Moss, S. (1984) The clarification and assessment of a method of psychotherapy. *British Journal of Psychiatry* 144, 567–80.

Gregg, V. (1986) *Introduction to Human Memory.* London. Routledge & Kegan Paul.

Haley, J. (1969) The art of being a failure as a therapist. *American Journal of Orthopsychiatry* 39, 691–5.

Hawton, K., Salkovskis, P.M., Kirk, J. & Clark, D.M. (1989) *Cognitive Behaviour Therapy for Psychiatric Problems. A Practical Guide.* Oxford. Oxford University Press.

Helfer, R.E. (1970) An objective comparison of the paediatric interviewing skills of freshmen and senior medical students. *Paediatrics* 45, 623–7.

Hobson, R.F. (1984) *The Heart of Psychotherapy.* London. Tavistock.

Hunt, J.M. & Marks-Maran, D.J. (1980) *Nursing Care Plans.* Aylesbury. H M+M.

Jacobson, E. (1938) *Progressive Relaxation.* Chicago. University of Chicago Press.

Jarvis, P. & Gibson, S. (1985) *The Teacher Practitioner in Nursing, Midwifery and Health Visiting.* London. Chapman & Hall.

Johnson, D.E. (1968) One conceptual model of nursing. *In* C.M.Beck *et al.* (1984) *Mental Health – Psychiatric Nursing: A Holistic Life-cycle Approach.* St Louis. Mosby.

Jung, J. (1968) *Verbal Learning.* New York. Holt, Rinehart & Winston.

Karoly, P. (1985) The assessment of pain: concepts and procedures. *In* P. Karoly (ed.) *Measurement Strategies in Health Psychology.* New York. Wiley.

Kazdin, A. (1982) *Single Case Research Designs.* New York. Oxford University Press.

Kendall, P.C. & Hollon, S.D. (1979) Cognitive-behavioral interventions: overview and current status. *In* P.C.Kendall & S.D.Hollon (Eds) *Cognitive-Behavioral Interventions. Theory, Research and Procedures.* New York. Academic Press.

King, I.M. (1971) *Towards a Theory of Nursing.* New York. Wiley.

Kirk, J. (1989) Cognitive-behavioural assessment. *In* K.Hawton, P.M.Salkovskis, J.Kirk,

& D.M.Clark (Eds) *Cognitive Behaviour Therapy for Psychiatric Problems. A Practical Guide.* Oxford. Oxford University Press.

Korsch, B.M., Gozzi, E.K. & Francis, V. (1968) Gaps in doctor–patient communications: 1. Doctor–patient interaction and patient satisfaction. *Paediatrics* 42, 855–71.

Lambert, M., deJulio, S. & Stein, D. (1978) Therapist interpersonal skills. *Psychological Bulletin* 83, 467–89.

Lang, P. (1971) The application of psychophysiological methods to the study of psychotherapy. *In* A.E.Bergin & S.L.Garfield (Eds) *Handbook of Psychotherapy and Behavior Change.* New York. Wiley.

Lazarus, A. (1973) Multimodal behaviour therapy: treating the BASIC I.D. *Journal of Nervous and Mental Disease* 156, 404–11.

Lethem, J., Slade, P.D., Troup, J.D.G. & Bentley, G. (1983) Outline of a fear-avoidance model of exaggarated pain perception – I. *Behaviour Research and Therapy* 21, 401–8.

Ley, P. (1976) Towards better doctor–patient communications. *In* A.E.Bennett (ed.) *Communication Between Doctors and Patients.* Oxford. Oxford University Press.

Ley, P. (1977) Psychological studies of doctor–patient communication. *In* S. Rachman (ed.) *Contributions to Medical Psychology.* Vol I. Oxford. Pergamon Press.

Ley, P. (1979) Improving clinical communication: effects of altering doctor–behaviour. *In* D.J.Oborne, M.M.Gruneberg & J.R.Eiser (Eds) *Research in Psychology and Medicine.* Vol II. London. Academic Press.

Ley, P. (1982) Satisfaction, compliance and communication. *British Journal of Clinical Psychology* 21, 241–54.

Ley, P. (1984) Psychological aspects of written information for patients. *In* S. Rachman (ed.) *Contributions to Medical Psychology.* Vol 3. Oxford. Pergamon Press.

Liberman, R.P., King, L.W., DeRisi, W.J. & McCann, M. (1975) *Personal Effectiveness: Guiding People to Assert Themselves and Improve Their Social Skills.* Champaign, Ill. Research Press.

Macguire, J. (1989) An approach to evaluating the introduction of primary nursing in an acute unit for the elderly – I. Principles and practice. *International Journal of Nursing Studies* 26, 3, 243–51.

Maguire, P. (1979) Teaching essential interviewing skills to medical students. *In* D.J.Oborne, M.M.Gruneberg & J.R.Eiser (Eds) *Research in Psychology and Medicine.* Vol. II. London. Academic Press.

Maguire, P. (1991) Managing difficult communication tasks. *In* R.Corney (ed.) *Developing Communication and Counselling Skills in Medicine.* London. Routledge.

Maguire, P. & Rutter, D.R. (1976) Teaching medical students to communicate. *In* A.E.Bennett (ed.) *Communication Between Doctors and Patients.* London. Oxford University Press.

Main, T.F. (1957) The ailment. *British Journal of Medical Psychology* 30, 128–45.

Marks, I.M. (1980) *Living With Fear.* New York. McGraw-Hill.

Marks, I.M. (1986) *Behavioural Psychotherapy: The Maudsley Pocket Book of Clinical Management.* Bristol. Wright.

Marks, I.M. (1987) *Fears, Phobias and Rituals.* New York. Oxford University Press.

Masson, J. (1990) *Against Therapy.* London. Fontana.

Mathews, A.M., Teasdale, J.D., Munby, M., Johnston, D. & Shaw, P. (1977) A home-based treatment program for agoraphobia. *Behavior Therapy* 8, 915–24.

Melzack, R. (1975) The McGill Pain Questionnaire: major properties and scoring methods. *Pain* 1, 277–99.

Newell, R. (1987) Treatment of irritable bowel syndrome by exposure in fantasy: a case report. *Behavioural Psychotherapy* 15, 381–7.

Newell, R. (1991) Disturbed body image: cognitive-behavioural formulation and treatment intervention. *Journal of Advanced Nursing* 16, 1400–5.

Newell, R. (1992) Anxiety, accuracy and reflection: the limits of professional development. *Journal of Advanced Nursing* 17, 1326–33.

Newell, R. & Dryden, W. (1991) Clinical problems: an introduction to the cognitive-behavioural approach. *In* W. Dryden & R. Rentoul (eds) *Clinical Problems: A Cognitive-behavioural Approach*. London. Routledge.

Newsome, A., Thorne, B. & Wylde, K. (1973) *Student Counselling in Practice*. London. University of London Press.

O'Leary, K.D. & Wilson, G.T. (1975) *Behaviour Therapy: Application and Outcome*. Englewood Cliffs, NJ. Prentice Hall.

Orne, M.T. (1962) On the social psychology of the psychological experiment: with particular reference to demand characteristics and their implications. *American Psychologist* 17, 776–800

Parkes, C.M. (1972) *Bereavement*. London. Tavistock.

Peck, D.F. & Shapiro, C.M. (1990) *Measuring Human Problems: A Practical Guide*. Chichester. Wiley.

Phillips, E.L. (1977) *Counseling and Psychotherapy: A Behavioral Approach*. New York. Wiley.

Popham, W.J., Eisner, E.W., Sullivan, H.J. & Tyler, L.L. (1969) *Instructional Objectives*. Chicago. Rand McNally.

Quinn, F.M. (1988) *The Principles and Practice of Nurse Education*. London. Chapman & Hall.

Rachman, S. (1977) Towards a new medical psychology. *In* S. Rachman (ed.) *Contributions to Medical Psychology*. Oxford. Pergamon Press.

Rachman, S.J. & Wilson, G.T. (1980) *The Effects of Psychological Therapy*. 2nd edn. Oxford. Pergamon.

Reilly, D. (1975) *Behavioural Objectives in Nursing: Evaluation of Learner Attainment*. New York. Appleton-Century-Crofts.

Richards, D.A. (1988) The treatment of a snake phobic by imaginal exposure. *Behavioural Psychotherapy* 16 (3), 207–16.

Richards, D.A. & McDonald, R. (1990) *Behavioural Psychotherapy: A Handbook for Nurses*. Oxford. Heinemann.

Rogers, C.R. (1951) *Client-Centred Therapy*. Boston. Houghton-Mifflin.

Rogers, C.R. (1957) The necessary and sufficient conditions of therapeutic personality change. *Journal of Consulting Psychology* 21, 95–103.

Rogers, M.E. (1980) A science of unitary man. *In* J.P. Riehl & C. Roy (eds) *Conceptual Models for Nursing Practice*. 2nd edn. New York. Appleton-Century-Crofts.

Roper, N., Logan, W.W. & Tierney, A.J. (1980) *The Elements of Nursing*. Edinburgh. Churchill Livingstone.

Russell, G. (1981) The current treatment of anorexia nervosa. *British Journal of Psychiatry* 138, 164–6.

Salkovskis, P.M. & Warwick, H.M.C. (1986) Morbid preoccupations, health anxiety and reassurance: a cognitive-behavioural approach to hypochondriasis. *Behaviour Research and Therapy* 24, 597–602.

Salkovskis, P.M., Jones, D.R.O. & Clark, D.M. (1986) Respiratory control of panic attacks: replication and extension with concurrent measurement of behaviour and pCO_2. *British Journal of Psychiatry* 148, 526–32.

Saylor, C.R. (1990) Reflection and nurse education: art, science and competency. *Nurse Educator* 15, 2, 8–11.

Schon, D.A. (1983) *The Reflective Practitioner: How Professionals Think in Action*. London. Temple Smith.

Schon, D.A. (1987) *Educating the Reflective Practitioner: Towards a New Design for Teaching and Learning in the Professions*. San Francisco. Jossey-Bass.

Shaffer, L.H. (1975) Multiple attention in continuous verbal tasks. *In* P.Rabbit & S. Dornic (eds) *Attention and Performance*. Vol 5. London. Academic Press.

Shapiro, M.B. (1961a) A method of measuring psychological changes specific to the individual psychiatric patient. *British Journal of Medical Psychology* 34, 151–5.

Shapiro, M.B. (1961b) The single case in fundamental psychological research. *British Journal of Medical Psychology* 34, 255–62.

Sommer, R. (1959) Studies in personal space. *Sociometry* 22, 247–60.

Stockwell, F. (1972) *The Unpopular Patient*. London. Royal College of Nursing.

Sundeen, S.J., Stuart, G.W., Rankin, E.A. DeS. & Cohen, S.A. (1989) *Nurse–Client Interaction: Implementing the Nursing Process*. St Louis. Mosby.

Sutherland, G., Newman, B. & Rachman, S.J. (1982) Experimental investigations of the relations between mood and unwanted intrusive cognitions. *British Journal of Medical Psychology* 55, 127–38.

Szasz, T. (1960) The myth of mental illness. *American Psychologist* 15, 113–18.

Thompson, J. (1984a) Communicating with patients. *In* R. Fitzpatrick, J. Hinton, S. Newman, G. Scambler & J. Thomson (eds) *The Experience of Illness*. London. Tavistock.

Thompson, J. (1984b) Compliance. *In* R. Fitzpatrick, J. Hinton, S. Newman, G. Scambler & J. Thomson (eds) *The Experience of Illness*. London. Tavistock.

Trower, P., Bryant, B. & Argyle, M. (1978) *Social Skills and Mental Health*. London. Methuen.

Vandecreek, L. & Angstadt, L. (1985) Client preferences and anticipations about counselor self-disclosure. *Journal of Counseling Psychology* 32, 206–14.

Walker, S.F. (1984) *Learning Theory & Behaviour Modification*. London. Methuen.

Walker, S.F. (1987) *Animal Learning*. London. Routledge & Kegan Paul.

Webb, C. (1983) Teaching for recovery from surgery. *In* J. Wilson-Barnett (ed.) *Patient Teaching*. Edinburgh. Churchill Livingstone.

Weiss, S.J. (1979) The language of touch. *Nursing Research* 28, 76–80.

Welford, A.T. (1976) *Skilled Performance: Perceptual and Motor Skills*. Glenville, Ill. Scott, Foreman & Co.

Williams, J.M.G., Watts, F.N., MacLeod, C. & Mathews, A. (1988) *Cognitive Psychology and Emotional Disorders*. Chichester. Wiley.

Wilson-Barnett, J. (1983) *Patient Teaching*. Edinburgh. Churchill Livingstone.

Wilson-Barnett, J. (1991) Providing relevant information for patients and their families. *In* R.Corney (ed.) *Developing Communication and Counselling Skills in Medicine*. London. Routledge.

Wittrock, M.C. (1989) Generative processes of comprehension. *Educational Psychologist* 24, 325–44.

Yule, W. & Hemsley, D. (1977) Single case method in medical psychology. *In* S. Rachman (ed.) *Contributions to Medical Psychology*. Oxford. Pergamon Press.

Author index

Subject index